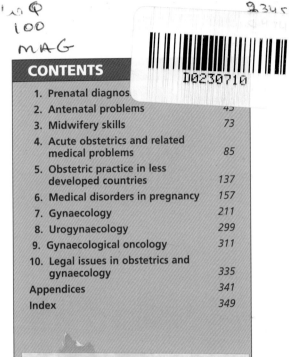

CONTENTS

Obstetrics and Gynaecology

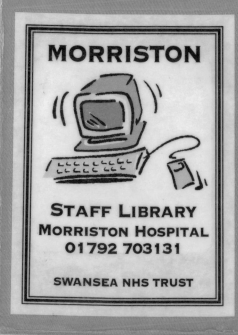

Commissioning Editor: Ellen Green
Development Editor: Hannah Kenner
Project Manager: David Fleming
Design Direction: Erik Bigland
Illustrators: Ian Ramsden and Jim Hope

CHURCHILL'S POCKETBOOKS

Obstetrics and Gynaecology

Brian Magowan MB ChB DCH MRCOG Dip Obs USS
Consultant Obstetrician and Gynaecologist, and
Head of Clinical Service
Borders General Hospital
Scotland, UK

THIRD EDITION

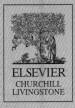

ELSEVIER
CHURCHILL
LIVINGSTONE

EDINBURGH LONDON NEW YORK OXFORD
PHILADELPHIA ST LOUIS SYDNEY TORONTO 2005

First edition 1997
Second edition 2000
This edition 2005

ISBN 0443101485
International Student Edition ISBN 0443101493

British Library Cataloguing in Publication Data
A catalogue record for this book is available from the British Library

Library of Congress Cataloging in Publication Data
A catalog record for this book is available from the Library of Congress

Note
Medical knowledge is constantly changing. Standard safety precautions must be followed, but as new research and clinical experience broaden our knowledge, changes in treatment and drug therapy may become necessary or appropriate. Readers are advised to check the most current product information provided by the manufacturer of each drug to be administered to verify the recommended dose, the method and duration of administration, and contraindications. It is the responsibility of the practitioner, relying on experience and knowledge of the patient, to determine dosages and the best treatment for each individual patient. Neither the Publisher nor the author assumes any liability for any injury and/or damage to persons or property arising from this publication.

The Publisher

CONTENTS

PREFACE

This edition, the third, has evolved at least as much from the second as it in turn evolved from the first. But whereas evolution is a gradual process, occurring in small quanta, it is exciting to see how much has changed in our specialty over such a short space of time. It is also humbling to see how much 'fact' has been reconsidered and revised in the light of excellent new research. 'It is unwise,' in the words of Mahatma Ghandi (1869-1948), 'to be too sure of one's own wisdom. It is healthy to be reminded that the strongest might weaken and the wisest might err'.

In addition to these revisions, new chapters have been added to highlight the importance of skilled midwifery, and to outline something of obstetric practice in less affluent parts of the world. The overall aim, however, is still to provide a useful and practical 'on-the-spot' reference text for medical staff, midwives, medical students and other health professionals.

Watching parents holding their new baby for the first time is a tremendous experience. It is a privilege to have been involved in some way with a successful birth, and those who have assisted may have feelings of pride and importance. When events go disastrously wrong, however, the feelings of dread and responsibility are often heavy to carry. Parents expect to return home with a healthy baby – they are counting on the doctor and midwife more than on anyone else before, and will remember their care for the rest of their lives. This care is up to you.

BM

STARTER POINTS

- As a junior doctor in obstetrics you will probably find yourself calling for seniors' support more often than in any previous post. This is good practice. In addition, do not hesitate to involve other specialists, particularly for medical or surgical problems or with acute labour ward obstetrics.
- Accept that most midwives are more experienced than junior doctors; listen hard to their opinions.
- When you walk into a labour room, look at the parents before looking at the CTG.
- If you have been involved in a delivery, do your best to see the mother at some stage in her postnatal stay. She will usually be delighted that you took the trouble and it often allows an opportunity to go over what happened.
- Time spent with the bereaved is very important for them and for you. Always allow the family to talk about the one they have lost (use the baby's name if one has been given).
- Beware of amateur scanning. Anyone can get a nice picture, but not everyone can see everything in the picture.
- Above all, always remember that it is often harder to do nothing than to do something.
- Despite the increasing application of scientific techniques, most of obstetric practice carries a large element of uncertainty. Think carefully, however, about how you personally will cope with this uncertainty. Will you become obsessively meticulous, never reassuring your patients for fear of losing your pride? Will you seek to blame others for your own imperfections? Or will you accept it as the inevitable, but exciting, unpredictability of an uncertain world? It is hoped that this book will provide a practical framework around which to build up a richness of personal experience.

ACKNOWLEDGEMENTS

I would like to thank the following for sharing their expertise in the preparation of this edition:

Sister Sarah Horan and Sister Lesley Rendell, The Borders General Hospital, Melrose
(Midwifery Skills)

Dr Susheel Vani, Research Registrar, New Royal Infirmary of Edinburgh, Edinburgh
(Obstetric Practice in Less Developed Countries)

Dr Alan Mathers, Consultant Obstetrician and Clinical Director, Princess Royal Maternity Hospital, Glasgow
(Acute Obstetrics)

Dr Philip Owen, Consultant Obstetrician and Gynaecologist, Princess Royal Maternity Hospital, Glasgow
(Gynaecology)

Dr Scott Fegan, Research Registrar, New Royal Infirmary of Edinburgh, Edinburgh
(Gynaecological Oncology)

Dr Ruth Richmond, Consultant Rheumatologist, The Borders General Hospital, Melrose
(Medical Disorders in Pregnancy)

Dr Roddy Campbell, Consultant Obstetrician and Gynaecologist, The Borders General Hospital, Melrose
(Medical Disorders in Pregnancy)

I would also like to thank Miss Marion McKenzie for her patient typing, photocopying, letter posting and support.

ABBREVIATIONS

αFP	α-fetoprotein		AV	atrioventricular
ABGs	arterial blood gases		AXR	abdominal X-ray
AC	abdominal circumference		AZT	zidovudine
ACE	angiotensin converting enzyme		BCG	Bacille–Calmette–Guérin
ACTH	adrenocorticotrophic hormone		BD	bis die (twice a day)
AD	autosomal dominant		BMI	body mass index
AF	atrial fibrillation		BP	blood pressure
AFI	amniotic fluid index		BPD	biparietal diameter
AGA	appropriate for gestational age		BSO	bilateral salpingo-oophorectomy
AIDS	autoimmune deficiency syndrome		BTS	blood transfusion service
AITP	autoimmune thrombocytopenia purpura		CAH	congenital adrenal hyperplasia
ANF	antinuclear factor		CCAM	congenital cystic adenomatoid malformation
AP	anteroposterior		CDH	congenital dislocated hip
APH	antepartum haemorrhage		CGMP	cyclic guanosine monophosphate
APTT	activated partial thromboplastin time		CHB	congenital heart block
AR	autosomal recessive		CHD	congenital heart disease
ARDS	adult respiratory distress syndrome		CHM	complete hydatidiform mole
ARF	acute renal failure		CI	contraindicated
ARM	artificial rupture of membranes		CIN	cervical intraepithelial neoplasia
ASAP	as soon as possible		CMV	cytomegalovirus
ASD	atrial septal defect		CNS	central nervous system
AST	aspartate transaminase			

COC	combined oral contraceptive		**ECV**	external cephalic version
CP	cerebral palsy		**ED**	every day
CPR	cardiopulmonary resuscitation		**EDD**	estimated date of delivery
CRP	C-reactive protein		**EDTA**	ethylenediamine tetra-acetic acid
CSF	cerebrospinal fluid			
CT	computerized tomography		**EEG**	electroencephalogram
CTG	cardiotocograph		**ELISA**	enzyme linked immunosorbent assay
CVP	central venous pressure		**EMD**	electromechanical dissociation
CVS	chorionic villus sampling		**ERPOC**	evacuation of retained products of conception
CXR	chest X-ray			
D&C	dilatation and curettage		**ESR**	erythrocyte sedimentation rate
DC	direct current		**ET**	endotracheal
DHAS	dehydro-epiandrosterone sulphate		**EUA**	examination under anaesthetic
DI	detrusor instability		**FA**	fetal anomaly
DIC	disseminated intravascular coagulation		**FBC**	full blood count
			FBS	fetal blood sample
			FFP	fresh frozen plasma
DKA	diabetic ketoacidosis		**FFTS**	feto-fetal transfusion sequence
DUB	dysfunctional uterine bleeding			
			FH	fetal heart
DVT	deep venous thrombosis		**FIGO**	International Federation of Gynaecologists and Obstetricians
ECG	electrocardiogram			
ECMO	extracorporeal membrane oxygenation		**FL**	femur length
			FNA	fine-needle aspiration

FSH	follicle stimulating hormone		**HDL**	high density lipoprotein
FTA	fluorescent treponemal antibody		**HDN**	haemolytic disease of the newborn
G&S	group and save serum		**HELLP**	haemolysis, elevated liver enzymes, low platelets
G6PD	glucose-6-phosphatase deficiency		**HIV**	human immunodeficiency virus
GA	general anaesthetic		**hMG**	human menopausal gonadotrophin
GFR	glomerular filtration rate		**HNPCC**	hereditary non-polyposis colorectal cancer
GI	gastrointestinal		**HOCM**	hypertrophic obstructive cardiomyopathy
GnRH	gonadotrophin releasing hormone		**HPO**	hypothalamopituitary – ovarian
GP	general practitioner			
GSI	genuine stress incontinence		**HPV**	human papilloma virus
GTN	gestational trophoblastic neoplasia		**HRT**	hormone replacement therapy
GTN	glyceryl trinitrate		**HSG**	hysterosalpingograph
GTT	glucose tolerance test		**HSV**	herpes simplex virus
GU	genitourinary		**HUS**	haemolytic uraemic syndrome
GUM	genitourinary medicine		**HVS**	high vaginal swab
HAART	highly active antiretroviral therapy		**IBD**	inflammatory bowel disease
H'CRIT	haematocrit		**IBS**	irritable bowel syndrome
Hb	haemoglobin			
HBV	hepatitis B virus		**ICSI**	intracytoplasmic sperm injection
hCG	human chorionic gonadotrophin			

ICU	intensive care unit		**LDH**	lactic dehydrogenase
IDDM	insulin dependent diabetes mellitus		**LDL**	low density lipoprotein
Ig	immunoglobulin		**LFTs**	liver function tests
IHD	ischaemic heart disease		**LH**	luteinizing hormone
IM	intramuscular		**LHRH**	luteinizing hormone releasing hormone
INR	international normalized ratio		**LLETZ**	large loop electrodiathermy excision of the transformation zone
IOL	induction of labour			
IPPV	intermittent positive pressure ventilation		**LMP**	last menstrual period
ISSHP	International Society for the Study of Hypertension in Pregnancy		**LMW**	low molecular weight
			LMWH	low molecular weight heparin
ISSVD	International Society for the Study of Vulval Diseases		**LW**	labour ward
			MAOIs	monoamine oxidase inhibitors
ITU	intensive treatment unit		**MAR**	mixed antibody reaction
IUCD	intrauterine contraceptive device		**MCH**	mean corpuscular haemoglobin
IUD	intrauterine death		**MCHC**	mean corpuscular haemoglobin concentration
IUGR	intrauterine growth restriction			
IV	intravenous		**MCV**	mean cell volume
IVF	in vitro fertilization		**MF**	multifactorial
IVU	intravenous urogram		**MI**	myocardial infarction
KCT	kaolin clotting time			
LA	local anaesthetic		**MMR**	mumps, measles and rubella
LB	live birth			
LCR	ligase chain reaction		**MMT**	mixed Müllerian tumour

MODS	multiple organ dysfunctional syndrome		**PCOS**	polycystic ovarian syndrome
MOM	multiples of the median		**PCR**	polymerase chain reaction
MRC	Medical Research Council		**PDA**	patent ductus arteriosus
MRI	magnetic resonance imaging		**PG**	prostaglandin
MS	multiple sclerosis		**PHM**	partial hydatidiform mole
MSU	midstream urine		**PID**	pelvic inflammatory disease
NGU	non-gonococcal urethritis		**PMB**	postmenopausal bleeding
NIDDM	non-insulin-dependent diabetes mellitus		**PMS**	premenstrual syndrome
NS	not significant		**PN**	postnatal
NSAIDs	non-steroidal anti-inflammatory drugs		**PO**	per os (orally)
			POG	Progress in Obstetrics and Gynaecology
NT	nuchal translucency			
NTD	neural tube defect		**POP**	progestogen-only pill
NYC	New York City		**PPH**	postpartum haemorrhage
OA	occipitoanterior			
OD	once daily		**PPROM**	preterm prelabour rupture of the membranes
OD45	optical density at 450 μm			
			PPV	positive predictive value
OP	occipitoposterior			
OT	occipitotransverse		**Prl**	prolactin
P	pulse		**PROM**	prelabour rupture of the membranes
PA	pernicious anaemia			
PCC	postcoital contraception		**PTE**	pulmonary thromboembolus
PCB	postcoital bleed		**PTR**	prothrombin ratio

PUVA	ultraviolet A with psoralen		**SIRS**	systemic inflammatory response syndrome
PV	per vaginam		**SLE**	systemic lupus erythematosus
QID	quarter in die (four times a day)		**SRM**	spontaneous rupture of the membranes
RBBB	right bundle branch block		**SSRI**	selective serotonin reuptake inhibitor
RCC	red cell concentrate		**stat**	statim (at once)
RCOG	Royal College of Obstetricians and Gynaecologists		**STD**	sexually transmitted disease
RCT	randomized controlled trial		**SVD**	spontaneous vertex delivery
RDS	respiratory distress syndrome		**SVT**	supraventricular tachycardia
RMI	risk of malignancy index		**T13**	trisomy 13
RR	relative risk		**T18**	trisomy 18
RUQ	right upper quadrant		**T21**	trisomy 21
SANDS	Stillbirth and Neonatal Death Society		**T4**	thyroxine
			TA	transabdominal
SB	stillbirth		**TAH**	total abdominal hysterectomy
SC	subcutaneously			
SCBU	special care baby unit		**TB**	tuberculosis
SFD	small for dates		**TBA**	traditional birth attendant
SGA	small for gestational age		**3TC**	lamivudine
			TCRE	transcervical resection of endometrium
SHBG	sex hormone binding globulin		**TED**	thromboembolic deterrant
SIDS	sudden infant death syndrome		**TFT**	thyroid function test

TIA	transient ischaemic attack	**VATER**	vertebral, anal, tracheal, oesophageal and renal
TID	ter in die (three times a day)		
TOP	termination of pregnancy	**VDRL**	venereal diseases reference laboratories
TORCH	toxoplasmosis, rubella, CMV, HSV	**VE**	vaginal examination
TPHA	*Treponema pallidum* haemagglutination	**VF**	ventricular fibrillation
		VIN	vulval intraepithelial neoplasia
TPN	total parenteral nutrition		
TSH	thyroid stimulating hormone	**VQ**	ventilation–perfusion
		VSD	ventricular septal defect
TV	transvaginal		
TVT	tension-free vaginal tape	**VT**	ventricular tachycardia
TZ	transitional zone	**VTE**	venous thromboembolism
U&E	urea and electrolytes	**VUR**	vesicoureteric reflux
uE3	unconjugated oestriol	**VZIG**	varicella zoster immunoglobulin
USS	ultrasound scan	**WCC**	white cell count
UTI	urinary tract infection	**WHO**	World Health Organization
VACTERL	vertebral, anal, cardiac, tracheal, oesophageal, renal and limb	**XL**	X-linked
		ZIG	zoster immunoglobulin
VAIN	vaginal intraepithelial neoplasia		

PRENATAL DIAGNOSIS

INTRODUCTION

Ideally, if the parents of a baby with a congenital anomaly can be seen by the same person at each clinic visit, it may be possible to ease some of the anxiety they will be feeling. If a serious problem does develop, do not be afraid to allow parents to contact you personally at the hospital – most do not and the point of contact will be a reassurance.

The finding of some 'abnormality' in pregnancy transforms what was previously an exciting and joyous event into an extremely worrying and distressing time. This remains true even when the potential risks are small: for example being recalled for invasive testing after abnormal screening or with the finding of a choroid plexus cyst on routine ultrasound scan. The very greatest of care should be taken in explaining any findings to parents. Tact, understanding and reassurance (if appropriate) are paramount. The advice we give parents is of such importance that it will frequently be necessary to involve senior members of the obstetrics team as well as members of other specialties, particularly paediatricians, surgeons and clinical geneticists. The details provided here are simplified versions of what are frequently complex diagnostic problems which sometimes have uncertain outcomes, and possession of this book is not an excuse to deny parents access to specialists in this field.

AIMS OF PRENATAL DIAGNOSIS

These aims are fourfold:

- the identification at an early gestation of abnormalities incompatible with survival, or likely to result in severe handicap, in order to prepare parents and offer the option of termination of pregnancy (the most common reason)
- the identification of conditions which may influence the timing, site or mode of delivery (rare)
- the identification of fetuses who would benefit from early paediatric intervention (rare)
- the identification of fetuses who may benefit from in utero treatment (very rare).

The first aim is usually the most controversial. Do not assume that all parents are going to request a termination of pregnancy even in the presence of lethal abnormality. Many couples opt to continue pregnancies even in the face of severe defects and express the view that they found it easier to cope with grief having held their child than having to face a termination. Others say that they were glad of the opportunity to terminate the pregnancy at an early stage and that they could not have coped with going on. More controversial still are the problems of chronic diseases with long-term handicap and long-term suffering for both the child and its parents. The parents themselves must decide what action they wish to take – it is they who will have to live with the decisions we place in front of them. It is our role to advise, guide and respect their final wishes, irrespective of our own personal views.

As thalamocortical connections do not develop until > 22 weeks, it is not possible for the fetus to feel pain before this gestation. Analgesia may be used for procedures > 24 weeks, but it is unlikely that there is fetal 'awareness' until 26 weeks.

NORMAL VIEWS FOR BPD, AC AND FL
(FIGS 1, 2, 3)

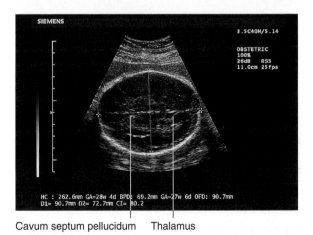

Cavum septum pellucidum   Thalamus

Fig. 1.1 Normal biparietal diameter. (Reproduced with permission from Siemens.)

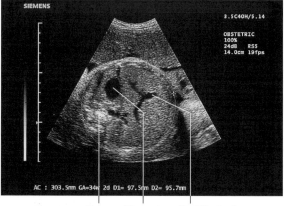

Spine   Stomach   Umbilical vein

Fig. 1.2 Normal abdominal circumference. (Reproduced with permission from Siemens.)

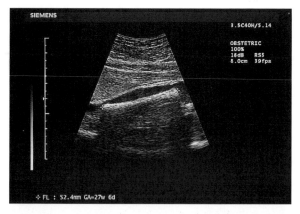

Fig. 1.3 Normal femur length. (Reproduced with permission from Siemens.)

SCREENING FOR FETAL ABNORMALITIES

Many structural anomalies can be seen on ultrasound scan, and many clinicians advocate that all mothers should be offered at least one detailed ultrasound at around 18–20 weeks or earlier. This has the advantage that previously unsuspected major or lethal anomalies (e.g.

spina bifida, renal agenesis) can be offered termination, and it also allows planned deliveries when conditions are present which may require early neonatal intervention (e.g. gastroschisis, transposition of the great arteries). Ultrasound scanning has the disadvantage, however, that many defects are not identified (it is likely that < 50% of cardiac defects are recognized in low risk pregnancies) and the false reassurance provided by this scan may become a source of parental resentment. Furthermore, some problem may be uncovered, for example one of the 'soft markers' (see below), the natural history of which is uncertain. This may generate unnecessary anxiety and increase the number of invasive diagnostic procedures (and thereby the loss rate) in otherwise healthy pregnancies.

Chromosomal abnormalities are much more difficult to identify on scan. While around half or two-thirds of fetuses with Down's syndrome will look normal at 18 weeks, most with Edward's and Patau's syndromes do show some abnormality, even though these abnormalities are often not specific or diagnostic. The two most commonly used screening tests for chromosomal abnormalities are measurement of the nuchal translucency at 11–14 weeks and the use of serum markers at ≥ 15 weeks.

NUCHAL TRANSPARENCY

Antenatal screening for Down's syndrome is possible by measuring the fetal nuchal translucency (NT) on ultrasound between 11–14 weeks (Fig. 1.4) and, ideally, also measuring the serum levels of free beta human chorionic gonadotrophin (β-hCG) and pregnancy associated plasma protein-A (PAPP-A). Combining the results of these tests allows the calculation of a 'chance' ratio, e.g. $1:50$ or $1:10\,000$ for carrying a fetus with Down's syndrome. Those with a risk above a certain value, say $1:300$, can then be offered an invasive diagnostic test in the form of either chorionic villus sampling (CVS) or amniocentesis. CVS may be carried out after 11 weeks' gestation and involves inserting a needle into the placenta and aspirating placental tissue for analysis. Amniocentesis can be carried out after 15 weeks' gestation and involves aspirating some of the amniotic fluid from around the baby, again under ultrasound guidance. Both these invasive procedures may cause miscarriage. The miscarriage rate for amniocentesis is around 0.5–1%. In very experienced hands, CVS may carry the same complication rate as amniocentesis at 15 weeks, but for most practitioners the risk is probably higher, at around 2–3%. Using the above screening method, and offering invasive testing to those with a risk greater than $1:300$ (i.e. around 5% of those

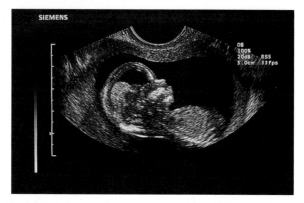

Fig. 1.4 Nuchal translucency measurement at 13 weeks (Reproduced with permission from Siemens.)

screened, depending on age), 90% of fetuses with Down's syndrome can be identified (BJOG 2003;110:281). It should be noted that increased NT is also a marker for structural defects (4% of those > 3 mm), particularly cardiac, diaphragmatic hernia, renal, abdominal wall and other more rare abnormalities. The overall survival for those with NT > 5 mm is ≈ 50%.

The choice between CVS and amniocentesis depends on more than just the gestation and the miscarriage rate. One per cent of those undergoing CVS will show mosaicism which is limited to the placenta and does not affect the fetus ('confined placental mosaicism'), but errors from this can be virtually eliminated if decisions are deferred until both the direct and culture results are available. This karyotypic discrepancy between fetus and placenta increases with increasing gestation. Results from both tests can be available within days of testing. Although diagnosis in the first trimester seems preferable to a second trimester diagnosis, there is work to show that psychological parental morbidity is independent of gestation, and indeed medical (TOP) may carry less psychological morbidity than surgical TOP (even if medical complications are higher).

SERUM SCREENING

Another screening method for chromosomal abnormality involves measuring levels of serum markers at 15+ weeks' gestation, particularly low levels of αFP, high hCG and low unconjugated oestriol. By correcting these for maternal weight and adjusting the results for maternal age, 70–80% of fetuses with Down's syndrome can be identified by carrying out an amniocentesis on around 5% of the screened population (Lancet 2003;361:835). The cut-off for recall is again set to a specified level (e.g. 1 : 250). As with NT screening, the pick-up rate is higher in older women, but the chance of being recalled with an elevated risk is also higher (Table 1.1). It is therefore not appropriate to advise women over the age of 35 years to have an amniocentesis based on age alone, as screening is more sensitive in the older age group.

This serum screening method can also be used to identify those with an open neural tube defect, particularly where there is no plan to carry out a routine detailed ultrasound scan. Those with levels greater than 2.0–2.5 multiples of the median can be selected for a detailed ultrasound scan. The test has a sensitivity of around 85% for neural tube detection. Maternal serum αFP may also be elevated following first-trimester bleeding, or with intrauterine death, twins, abdominal wall defects, congenital nephrosis, Turner's syndrome, epidermolysis bullosa, rhesus disease and renal agenesis. It is important to bear in mind that, even if the ultrasound scan is normal, an elevated αFP is still a marker for later pre-eclampsia or intrauterine growth restriction (Table 1.2) and there is evidence that Doppler studies may help to identify this group. If the αFP and hCG are both raised, at least 60% of pregnancies are likely to have some complication.

TABLE 1.1 Serum screening for Down's syndrome on varying age groupings

Age	Sensitivity (i.e. number of cases picked up)	Recalled
< 25	35%	2%
25–29	40%	3%
30–34	54%	7%
35	⎫	13%
36	⎪	19%
37	⎬ 76%	19%
38	⎪	26%
39	⎭	32%
40–44	93%	44%
> 45	> 99%	85%

TABLE 1.2 Associations following raised αFP and normal ultra-sound scan			
	Extremely SGA (< 2.2nd centile)	SGA (< 10th centile)	Preterm delivery (AGA)
↑ αFP (> 2.5 MOM)	9.4% (RR 4.5)	27% (RR 2.7)	14% (RR 2.4)
↑ hCG	4.4% (RR 2.1)	15% (RR 1.5)	NS
↑ αFP + hCG	24% (RR 10.9)	38%	47% (RR 3.0)

ANEUPLOIDY

SYNDROMES

Trisomy 21 (Down's syndrome)

The overall incidence is 1 : 650 LBs, but the individual incidence is dependent on maternal age. Most Down's syndrome children, however, are born to younger mothers as they have proportionately more babies. Although walking, language and self-care skills are usually attained, independence is rare. There is mental retardation (with a mean IQ around 50) and an association with CHD (particularly AV canal defects, VSD, PDA, ASD primum and Fallot's tetralogy). GI atresias are common, and there is early dementia with similarities to Alzheimer's disease. Twenty per cent die before the age of 1 year and 45% reach 60 years old.

Incidence

20 years 1 : 2000	38 years 1 : 180
30 years 1 : 900	40 years 1 : 100
35 years 1 : 350	44 years 1 : 40
36 years 1 : 240	

Overall, 95% of cases are due to non-dysjunction, with translocation 14 : 21 accounting for 2%, other translocations 2% and mosaicism 1%. Half of the translocations occur de novo. The recurrence risk for non-dysjunction is an additional 0.75% above the background risk. If there is a 14 : 21 translocation in the mother the recurrence risk is 1 : 10, and 1 : 50 if this translocation is present in the father.

Trisomy 18 (Edward's syndrome)

Incidence 1 : 2500 LBs. Most are due to non-dysjunction. The baby has IUGR, a small elongated head (strawberry shaped on USS), severe mental retardation, rocker bottom feet and an increased incidence of

GI and renal anomalies. CHD is almost invariable (usually VSD, ASD or PDA), and overlapping fingers and flexion deformities may also be seen. Overall, 50% die before the age of 2 months and 90% before the end of the first year.

Trisomy 13 (Patau's syndrome)

Incidence 1 : 5000 LBs. Overall, 75% of cases are due to non-dysjunction. There is IUGR, severe mental retardation and an increased incidence of cleft palate, GI atresias and holoprosencephaly. In 80% of cases there is CHD. The majority of children die before the age of 3 months, and rarely survive after the age of 1 year. A very small number may survive for years.

Triploidy

Fetuses rarely survive to birth and there is no survival beyond the neonatal period.

XO (Turner's syndrome)

Incidence 1:3000 LBs. Overall, 60% of cases are pure XO, ≥15% are mosaics (usually XO/XX) and the rest are deletions, rings or isochromosomes of Xq or Xp. The incidence is increased with increasing paternal age and decreased with increasing maternal age. Antenatally there may be a cystic hygroma ± generalized oedema and cardiac defects. Postnatally there may be short stature, cubitus valgus, coarctation of the aorta, a bicuspid aortic valve, streak gonads and, only occasionally, a lowered IQ. A small proportion may be fertile (particularly mosaics and deletions), although the incidence of premature ovarian failure is high. The risks of pregnancy loss and karyotypic abnormalities in those with XO are also greater.

XXX

1 : 1000 LBs. The incidence is increased with increasing maternal age. The phenotype and fertility are normal and the abnormality frequently goes unnoticed. There is, however, an increased risk of sex chromosome abnormalities (≈ 4%) and premature menopause in the offspring.

XXX + (i.e. more than three X chromosomes)

This is rare. Dysmorphism and mental retardation are common, as is menstrual dysfunction. The individual may be fertile.

XXY (Klinefelter's syndrome)

1 : 700–2000 LBs. The incidence is increased with advanced maternal age. The individual is phenotypically a tall male, with an occasionally

reduced IQ, sparse facial hair and gynaecomastia. It is the commonest single cause of male hypogonadism and is usually diagnosed in the investigation of male infertility. There is an association with hypothyroidism, diabetes and asthma. Azoospermia is the rule.

XYY

1:700 LBs. The incidence of this is not associated with maternal age. The IQ and fertility are usually normal and the suggestion of increased impulsive behaviour may be biased by the population sampled. Individuals are usually tall. The risk of sex chromosome abnormalities in offspring is $\approx 4\%$.

Apparently balanced rearrangements (translocations or inversions)

If found at amniocentesis it is essential to karyotype the parents. If one parent has the translocation and is phenotypically normal, it is likely that the fetus will be phenotypically normal as well. Possible pregnancy outcomes when one parent carries a balanced translocation are of a normal karyotype, a fetus with a balanced translocation (phenotypically like its parent as above), and a fetus with an unbalanced translocation. In general the smaller the section of chromosome involved in the unbalanced translocation, the greater the likelihood of a fetus surviving to term, often with problems. Larger sections of chromosome are associated with in-utero loss. If a fetal translocation has been found to occur de novo, the overall risk of phenotypic abnormality is in the order of 10% but as some chromosomal re-arrangements are normal population variants, genetic advice should always be sought.

Unbalanced chromosomal structural abnormalities

Many abnormalities are well characterized, but it is often difficult to be specific. Parental karyotyping is required and genetic advice should be sought. Mental impairment is common, and physical abnormality is possible.

SOFT MARKERS

These are structural features found on USS that in themselves are not usually a problem, but which may be pointers to aneuploidy. They are found in $\approx 5\%$ of all pregnancies in the second trimester and are the cause of a lot of parental anxiety. Assignment of risk for aneuploidy is fraught with difficulty as adequate data from low-risk pregnancies are very limited. If isolated, the risk of chromosomal problems is low, and any risk assessment needs to take maternal age and any other prenatal test results into account. If more than one soft marker is found, or if there are any other structural defects, the risk is very much higher. The more subtle markers (clinodactyly, sandal gap, polydactyly, etc.) are not discussed here. The use of soft markers to screen a low risk population is not appropriate as there is a large increase in invasive testing for virtually no increased pick-up over and above prior testing. A good case can be made for not reporting isolated soft markers in an already screened population.

Borderline ventriculomegaly

The normal ventricle measures 6.6 ± 1.2 mm; 10 mm is $> 3SD$. Ventriculomegaly is said to be present if one or both of the ventricles measures > 10 mm. The risk of aneuploidy is $\approx \times 1.5$ the baseline age-related risk.

Choroid plexus cysts

The choroid plexus may demonstrate small cysts *with hyperechoic capsules* (up to about 10 mm in diameter) in early pregnancy. These are present in 1% of all 18-week scans, are often bilateral, are thought to be developmental in origin and usually disappear by 24 weeks' gestation. There is a small association with T18 and T13, and probably no association with T21. If other abnormalities are present the risk of aneuploidy is high. It is important to consider whether invasive testing is appropriate in the presence of an otherwise normal scan as long-term survival of T18 is so exceptional. Both size and resolution are unrelated to karyotype risk.

Echogenic bowel

Echogenic bowel is a midtrimester finding that occurs in less than 1% of pregnancies, although the incidence of reporting varies widely between different observers. The bowel is bright, being similar to the spine/ribs in echogenicity. There is a small association with aneuploidy ($< 3\%$), cystic fibrosis ($0–13\%$) and perinatal death ($\approx 10\%$). Parents should be tested for cystic fibrosis mutations but decisions about fetal karyotyping should depend on other findings and tests. A normal outcome can be anticipated in most cases overall, and in the majority of whom hyperechogenic bowel is an isolated finding.

Echogenic foci

There is a moving echogenic focus (or 'golf ball') within either one or both cardiac ventricles which has no obvious anatomically associated structure, but may represent papillary microcalcification (Fig. 1.5). The incidence is $\approx 3\%$. Structural heart disease should be excluded

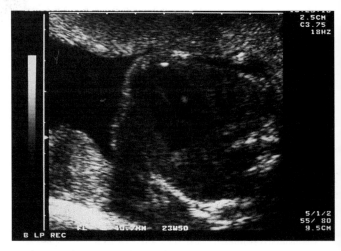

Fig. 1.5 Left ventricular echogenic focus in an otherwise normal 4-chamber view at 20 weeks' gestation → normal outcome.

(see below). There may be a slightly increased risk of T21, but this risk is probably less than 1% with isolated lesions.

Renal pelvic dilatation

This is defined as a dilatation of > 4 mm before 33 weeks and > 7 mm after 33 weeks (Fig. 1.6). The T21 and T18 risk is increased approximately 1.5-fold over age-related risk alone. If serum or NT screening for aneuploidy has already been carried out, however, almost certainly no further action is required. There is also an association with postnatal reflux, UTI and renal scarring (see p. 23).

STRUCTURAL DISORDERS

CONGENITAL HEART DISEASE

This is the commonest congenital malformation in children and affects about 5–8:1000 live births. Approximately 2–3 of these 8 are severe malformations. Of defects diagnosed antenatally, about 15% are associated with aneuploidy, most commonly T18 and T21.

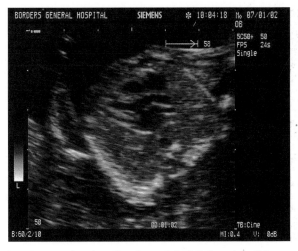

Fig. 1.6 A normal aortic outflow view excludes Fallot's tetralogy. If the pulmonary outflow is also normal, transposition of the great arteries can also be excluded.

Antenatal diagnosis

Certain groups carry a greater risk of CHD particularly in those:

- with extracardiac anomalies (20%)
- with a CHD in either parent (particularly the mother) or a sibling (2–6%)
- with diabetes mellitus (3%, although possibly less with better diabetic control in the first trimester)
- who have been exposed to teratogens, particularly lithium and anticonvulsants
- with fetal arrhythmias, particularly CHB (P < 100 bpm)
- with non-immune hydrops fetalis
- with increased NT between 11 and 14 weeks.

The four-chamber view of the heart can be used to identify 25–40% of all major abnormalities (Fig. 1.5). In addition, viewing the aorta and pulmonary artery increases the sensitivity of picking up structural abnormalities to ≥ 60% (Fig. 1.6). At 18 weeks most of the major connections can be seen, but high-risk pregnancies should be rescanned at 22–26 weeks to identify more minor defects.

Scanning fetal hearts

Check that the heart is on the left and obtain a four-chamber view. Deviation of the cardiac axis to the left (> 75° from midline) and the right (< 25°) is strongly associated with structural abnormality. The heart should occupy approximately one-third of the thorax and have a normal, regular rhythm (use M-mode if necessary). Look at contractility and check for a pericardial effusion. The right ventricle lies behind the sternum, and the left atrium (with its connecting pulmonary veins) is in front of the descending thoracic aorta. Both ventricles should be the same size (one small ventricle suggests left- or right-sided hypoplasia), and the interventricular septum, when viewed at 90° to the direction of scanning, should be intact (i.e. no VSDs). The right ventricle has a moderator band at its apex and the tricuspid valve is inserted a little more towards the apex than the mitral valve. While the valves should close synchronously, they should be seen to move independently.

By inclining the transducer more cephalad, it is possible to see the aortic outflow from the left ventricle in the direction of the right fetal shoulder and, further cephalad, the pulmonary artery. This arises from the right ventricle and crosses the aorta at approximately 90° on its way posteriorly (a pulmonary artery parallel to the aorta suggests transposition of the great arteries). The anterior wall of the aorta should be continuous with the interventricular septum (discontinuity suggests VSD or endocardial cushion defect) and should not override the interventricular septum (suggests Fallot's tetralogy).

Arrhythmias

Irregular Usually premature atrial contractions (extrasystolic beats, dropped beats). Ventricular ectopic beats are very rare. Only 1–2% proceed to a tachyarrhythmia, and the risk of structural heart disease is also only 1–2%.

Bradycardia Usually congenital heart block (atrial movement appears independent of the ventricle). Exclude maternal anti Ro or La antibodies (see p. 161). If there is abnormal anatomy, the prognosis is very poor. If structurally normal, the prognosis is variable:

- if hydropic, < 50% survive
- if not, almost always OK
- if FH rate decreases or is < 50 bpm the prognosis is less good.

Postnatal pacing may be required and there is a risk of later cardiomyopathy. In utero treatment by maternal administration of steroids has occasionally been associated with resolution; the benefit of chronotropic agents is very uncertain.

Tachyarrhythmias Almost always SVT with a rate of 220–240 bpm. Atrial flutter/fibrillation is less common and ventricular tachycardia is only rarely reported. The presence of hydrops is associated with a poorer prognosis. Diagnosis and management should be coordinated in a tertiary referral unit. Treatment options are limited. Both digoxin and flecainide have both been used successfully, but are potentially toxic to the mother. You should involve fetal medicine specialists.

CRANIOSPINAL DEFECTS (MF)

Neural tube defects (see also Screening, p. 6)

- *Anencephaly*: the skull vault and cerebral cortex are absent.
- *Spina bifida*:
  — meningocele: dura and arachnoid mater bulge through the defect
  — myelomeningocele: the central canal of the cord is exposed.
- *Encephalocele*: there is a bony defect in the cranial vault through which a dura mater sac (± brain tissue) protrudes.

Spina bifida and anencephaly make up more than 95% of NTDs. There is wide geographical variation in births, with a higher incidence in Scotland and Ireland (3 : 1000), and a lower incidence in England (2 : 1000), the USA, Canada, Japan and Africa (< 1 : 1000). There is good evidence that the overall incidence has fallen over the past 15 years (independent of any screening programmes).

Recurrence risk is:

- with 1 affected sibling,   1 : 25
- with 2 or more affected siblings,   1 : 10
- with 1 affected parent,   1 : 25.

Anencephaly The infant is either stillborn or, if liveborn, will usually die shortly after birth (although some may survive for several days).

Spina bifida The spine can be viewed by ultrasound in three planes to assess the type and level of any deficit (Fig. 1.7). Hydrocephalus occurs in about 90% of fetuses with spina bifida and carries a much poorer prognosis than spina bifida alone. Markers for spina bifida (which are 99% sensitive) include blunting of the sinciput (the lemon sign, Fig. 1.8), a banana-shaped cerebellum (Arnold–Chiari malformation) and an absent cerebellum (Fig. 1.9). Those with myelomeningoceles usually have abnormal lower limb neurology, and many have hydrocephalus. In addition to immobility and mental retardation there may be problems with UTI, bladder dysfunction, bowel dysfunction, and social and sexual isolation. Around 90% are handicapped and 30% live to 5 years of age.

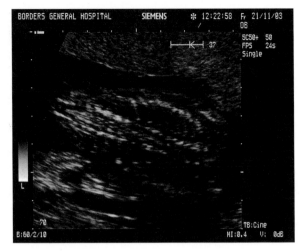

Fig. 1.7 Coronal view of spina bifida with dysraphism of the thoracolumbar vertebral bodies.

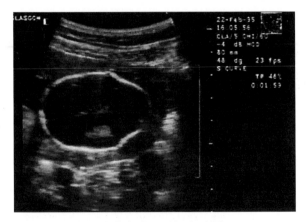

Fig. 1.8 Lemon-shaped skull of a fetus with spina bifida.

Encephalocele This may be occipital or frontal. Isolated meningoceles carry a good prognosis, whereas those with microcephaly secondary to brain herniation carry a very poor prognosis. As more than 95% of encephaloceles are closed defects, the maternal serum αFP level is usually normal.

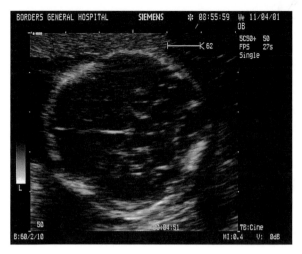

Fig. 1.9 A normal cerebellum – spina bifida is very unlikely.

Prevention

The MRC Vitamin Study Group (1991) showed that folate 4 mg/day PO taken from before conception reduced the recurrence risk of NTDs in those who had had an affected child previously. A preconceptual prophylactic dose of 400 µg/day PO for all pregnant women may be more physiological, and use of this dose is supported by earlier studies. There are, at present, no known teratogenic effects of folate.

Microcephaly

Most microcephalies are MF, but a few are AR. The head circumference is three standard deviations below the expected value compared to the rest of the measurements (e.g. abdominal circumference, femur length). The children are frequently mentally retarded, often severely. In general, the smaller the head the worse the prognosis, *but children have developed normally despite very small head circumferences*. The condition may occur following infection (particularly rubella), as part of a multiple malformation syndrome, or secondary to some other teratogen, but in most cases the cause is never established. In the absence of a known cause, the recurrence risk is 1 : 10. The diagnosis requires serial ultrasound scanning and is frequently not made until at least 24 weeks' gestation. As scanning after this stage is often not routine, many babies with microcephaly are missed prenatally.

Ventriculomegaly

Ventriculomegaly may be taken as a lateral ventricular atrium measurement of > 10 mm (Fig. 1.10). The head is usually normal sized. Hydrocephaly may be taken as further dilatation with thinning and 'dangling' of the dependent choroid plexus, and head size may (but does not necessarily) increase above centiles in later pregnancy.

Ventriculomegaly has a 30% association with spina bifida (see above). Those cases not associated with spina bifida may occur secondary to obstruction, usually at the aqueduct of Sylvius (with a normal 4th ventricle) or at the foraminae of Luschka and Magendi (the Dandy–Walker malformation); the latter carries a poor prognosis (note that there are variants of this condition). Rare forms of ventriculomegaly include holoprosencephaly (absent cavum septum pellucidum and a single cerebral ventricle – associated with T13) and agenesis of the corpus callosum (absent cavum septum pellucidum, 3rd ventricle dilatation and separation of the anterior horns of the lateral ventricles), both of which carry a very poor prognosis. There is also an association with chromosomal disorders, particularly if severe and in the presence of other abnormalities, although idiopathic borderline ventriculomegaly (10–12 mm) carries only a small risk of aneuploidy.

The prognosis of isolated ventriculomegaly is generally good unless the condition is progressive or severe. The prognosis is generally poor when other abnormalities are present. The recurrence

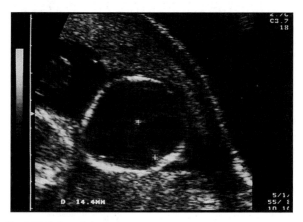

Fig. 1.10 Hydrocephalus.

risk for isolated hydrocephalus is about 1 : 30, but the much rarer sex-linked aqueduct stenosis carries a 1 : 4 risk of recurrence (1 : 2 if the fetus is already known to be male).

GASTROINTESTINAL DISORDERS

Abdominal wall defects

These may present because of an elevated maternal serum αFP.

Exomphalos (Fig. 1.11) This occurs following failure of the gut to return to the abdominal cavity at 8 weeks' gestation and results in a defect through which the peritoneal sac protrudes. This may contain both intestines and liver. There are chromosomal abnormalities in 30% (especially T18), and 10–50% have other lesions, particularly cardiac and renal. There is also an association with ectopia vesicae and ectopia cardia. If the exomphalos is isolated (i.e. there are no other structural abnormalities), the chromosomes are normal and there is no bowel atresia or infarction, the prognosis is good (> 80% long-term survival). The sac rarely ruptures at vaginal delivery. There is an association with Beckwith–Wiedmann syndrome (see p. 31).

Gastroschisis (Fig. 1.12)
This is commoner than exomphalos. The abdominal wall defect is usually to the right and below the insertion of the umbilical cord. Small

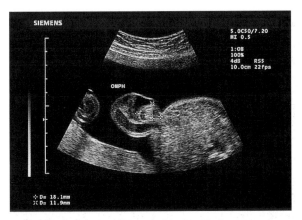

Fig. 1.11 A small exomphalos. (Reproduced with permission from Siemens.)

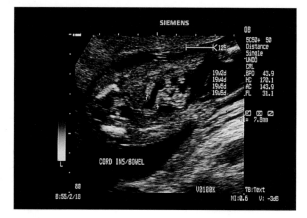

Fig. 1.12 Gastroschisis. (Reproduced with permission from Siemens.)

bowel (without a peritoneal covering) protrudes and floats free in the peritoneal fluid. Gut atresias and cardiac lesions occur in 20% of cases, but the association with chromosomal abnormality is very small (probably < 1%). The prognosis is good if the bowel is viable, although 10% of cases end in stillbirth despite apparently normal growth. Gut dilatation may be associated with bowel obstruction or ischaemia, but is not directly linked to prognosis. These babies are usually SFD and require very close surveillance. The recurrence risk is < 1%.

Bowel obstruction (MF)
Incidence 1 : 12 000 LBs. These are probably secondary to a vascular insult in early fetal life. There are multiple distended loops of bowel. The prognosis depends on the site of obstruction, the more distal carrying the better prognosis.

Duodenal atresia (MF)
Incidence 1 : 7000 LBs. The stomach and proximal duodenum distend to give the classic ultrasound double-bubble appearance and there is polyhydramnios. This may not be apparent on the 18-week scan, but is usually present by 25 weeks. There are other congenital malformations in 50%, including bowel, kidney and skeletal abnormalities. In 30% of cases there is T21. Jejunal atresia produces a triple-bubble appearance.

Echogenic bowel

See page 11.

Oesophageal atresia (MF)

Incidence 1 : 3000 LBs. The oesophagus is not readily seen on ultrasound, but the absence of a stomach bubble in the presence of polyhydramnios should raise the possibility of this diagnosis. In 90% of cases, however, there is a tracheo-oesophageal fistula which allows stomach filling, and the stomach bubble is present. There is an association with aneuploidy in 15%, and also with cardiac defects.

GENITOURINARY ABNORMALITIES

Renal cystic disease

Isolated cysts arising from the substance of the kidney are rare, and only become significant if they are so large that they prevent a vaginal delivery. It may not be possible to establish a precise diagnosis antenatally.

Renal dysplasia

Multicystic dysplastic kidneys (sporadic inheritance) The kidneys have large discrete non-communicating cysts with a central, more solid core

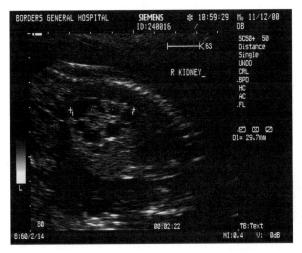

Fig. 1.13 Multicystic dysplastic kidney.

and are thought to follow early developmental failure (Fig. 1.13) or outflow obstruction. If the cysts affect only one kidney, the other is normal, and there is adequate liquor, the prognosis is good. If the cysts are bilateral and the liquor is reduced, the prognosis is poor.

Polycystic kidney disease

Adult polycystic kidney disease (AD) The corticomedullary junction is accentuated and the condition is relatively benign, often not producing symptoms until the fifth decade of life. Many individuals have ultrasonically normal kidneys at birth. There are at least two genes on different chromosomes, however, so that DNA studies are only possible in families with multiple affected members.

Infantile polycystic kidney disease (AR) There is a wide range of expression, with the size of cysts ranging from microscopic to several millimetres across. Both kidneys are affected, and there may also be cysts present in the liver and pancreas. Ultrasound features of oligohydramnios, empty bladder and large symmetrical bright kidneys (Fig. 1.14) may not develop until later in pregnancy. Check for occipital encephalocele. If there is survival beyond the neonatal period, there may be later problems with raised BP and progressive renal failure. Long-term survival is rare.

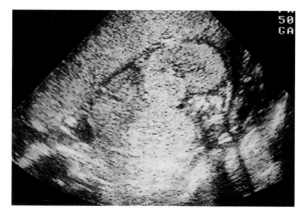

Fig. 1.14 Infantile polycystic kidney disease with anhydramnios at 26 weeks → intrauterine demise 2 weeks later.

Spine L. kidney L. renal pelvis

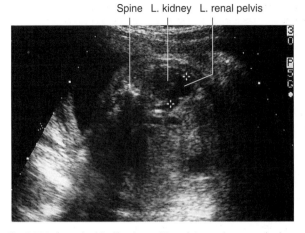

Fig. 1.15 Left renal pelvic dilatation at 33 weeks' gestation → resolved postnatally.

Obstruction

Urinary tract obstruction occurs at three main sites, as described below.

Pyelectasis (Fig. 1.15) This may be unilateral (79–90%) or bilateral. It is probably caused by a neuromuscular defect at the junction of the ureter and the renal pelvis, which presents with increasing pelvic dilatation in the presence of a normal ureter. The cortical thickness is usually well preserved, but later ultrasound review can be used to monitor the cortical thickness (increased echogenicity and hydroureter carry a poorer prognosis). There is no indication for induction of labour. As there is an association with postnatal UTIs and reflux nephropathy, it is reasonable to start all neonates on prophylactic antibiotics and arrange postnatal radiological follow-up (e.g. USS at 1–4 weeks, depending on severity, ± later micturating cystourethrogram). Even in those with mild dilatation (> 5 and < 10 mm) there is VUR in 10–20%, although only a small proportion require surgery. Vesicoureteric junction obstruction can also occur.

Posterior urethral valves Folds of mucosa at the bladder neck prevent urine leaving the bladder. The fetus is usually male, there is often oligohydramnios, and on ultrasound there are varying degrees of renal dysplasia. There is a chromosomal abnormality in 7% of isolated defects and in one-third of those with other abnormalities. If the chromosomes are normal, the obstruction is severe and urinary electrolytes are normal, it is possible to insert a pigtail shunt between the bladder and amniotic cavity. This may relieve the obstruction, but the long-term prognosis is still poor as the renal damage may not be reversible.

Urethral stenosis There is usually marked oligohydramnios with dilatation of the urinary bladder, often with bilateral dysplastic kidneys. The outcome is usually fetal demise, but pigtail catheter insertion has been used with some success.

Potter's syndrome (MF – sporadic)

Incidence 1 : 10 000 LBs. Bilateral renal agenesis is associated with extreme oligohydramnios and leads to the Potter's sequence of pulmonary hypoplasia (see p. 26) and limb deformity. The condition is lethal (and indeed severe mid-trimester oligohydramnios from any cause carries a relatively poor prognosis). Fetal ultrasound diagnosis is problematic because the low liquor level makes visualization difficult; transvaginal scanning and fluid installation are of help. There may be associated cardiac abnormalities. Adrenal glands can be mistaken for kidneys (in the absence of kidneys, the adrenals expand to fill the space). Serial scanning over a few hours to look for bladder filling is important (evidence of no renal function). This also helps to avoid confusion with ectopic kidneys. Renal arteries (as seen with Doppler) are only present if kidneys are present (although the presence of a kidney does not mean that it is functioning). The recurrence risk is approximately 3%, although AD forms with variable penetrance have been described.

HAEMOGLOBIN VARIANTS AND THALASSAEMIA

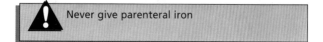

⚠ Never give parenteral iron

Haemoglobin is composed of four subunits, each made up of a globin chain and a haem component. Normal adult haemoglobin is made up of 2 α- and 2 β-globin chains. Disorders affecting the structure or synthesis of these chains are known as haemoglobinopathies. Screening may be targeted, based on ethnic background, but Caucasians may occasionally be carriers.

Disorders of globin structure

Haemoglobin structural variants result from a genetically determined chemical alteration in the globin molecule. There are many different pathological types, of which sickle-cell disease, a β-chain variant due to a single constant mutation, is the commonest.

Sickle-cell disease (AR)

This presents after the age of 6 months and, although 25% die before the age of 5 years, 50% survive to the age of 40. 'Crises', which may be precipitated by infection, dehydration, cold, hypoxia and stasis, affect joints, the back, long bones and spleen. In pregnancy there is an increased risk of pulmonary embolism and renal infarction. There is also a high fetal loss rate and increased chance of IUGR and prematurity. Maintain hydration, treat infection aggressively and transfuse only if the Hb is much lower than usual for that patient (and never to > 10 g/dl). Exchange transfusions should only be for those who are severely unwell. HbSC is a milder variant with near normal haemoglobin. Prenatal diagnosis is possible after parental testing, using either CVS or amniocentesis.

Sickle cell trait

Heterozygotes who carry the HbS mutation on one chromosome 16 have this trait. There are no clinical problems in this condition, and indeed there is some protection against the effects of falciparum malarial infection. Forty percent of haemoglobin on electrophoresis is HbS, with HbA2 comprising 3% and the remainder being HbA1. The MCV and Hb are normal.

Disorders of globin synthesis

Thalassaemia results from a genetically determined imbalanced production of one of the globin chains. α-Thalassaemia affects α-globin chains while β-thalassaemia affects β-globin chains. α-Globin is coded for by two genes on chromosome 16, while β-globin is coded for by one gene on chromosome 11. Those with an MCV < 76 fl or MCH < 27 pg should be considered for further investigation. If positive, screen the other parent. There are many different genetic defects with differing prognoses and DNA analysis is important.

β-Thalassaemia

β-Thalassaemia minor. This is loss of function of one β-globin gene, with the tendency to anaemia corrected with oral $FeSO_4$ and folate. The HbA2 is 4–6%, with a slightly elevated HbF.

β-Thalassaemia major (Cooley's anaemia) Loss of function of two β-globin genes gives rise to this condition. There is increased iron uptake (despite excess iron stores), anaemia and progression to death without transfusions. There are also later problems with endocrine failure (including secondary sexual development), osteoporosis, haemosiderosis and cardiac failure. Transfusions suppress endogenous haemopoiesis, preventing skeletal deformity from marrow overgrowth (Hep C infection is now common). Consistent chelation therapy reduces problems of iron toxicity, and hydroxyurea is also used. Pregnancy may be possible following ovulation induction in those with good cardiac function. Marrow transplant is possible. The HbF is 50–100% on electrophoresis.

α-Thalassaemia

HbH disease This is loss of function of three α-globin genes. There is mild anaemia, the life expectancy is normal and treatment is with oral folate. β4 Tetramers form 5–30% of the haemoglobin on electrophoresis.

Bart's hydrops This is loss of all four α-globin genes. The hydropic fetus is non-viable, and the pregnancy is associated with an increased incidence of eclampsia and obstructed labour. Treatment is by termination of pregnancy.

LUNG DISORDERS

Pulmonary hypoplasia

This occurs most commonly as a consequence of oligohydramnios secondary to very preterm prelabour membrane rupture, Potter's syndrome (see p. 24), or diaphragmatic hernia (see below). Attempts to predict lung function based on linear measurements, chest circumference, lung volume or the presence of breathing movements have been disappointing.

Diaphragmatic hernia

Incidence 1 : 5000 LBs. Stomach, colon and even spleen enter the chest through a defect in the diaphragm, usually on the left. The heart is pushed to the right and the lungs become hypoplastic. The incidence of aneuploidy is 15–30% and there is an association with NTDs, CHD and renal and skeletal abnormalities. The overall survival of those diagnosed antenatally is ≈ 20%, with a better prognosis for isolated left-sided herniae. Polyhydramnios, mediastinal shift and left ventricular compression are poor antenatal prognostic factors.

Increased nuchal translucency is also an adverse prognostic feature. For those who reach the stage of theatre, the survival rate is > 80%. Neither the use of ECMO or nitric oxide has improved the prognosis. The chance of recurrence is approximately 2%, although there are occasional X-linked forms. New experimental therapeutic strategies include the use of a guided indwelling balloon to obstruct the fetal trachea in utero, allowing lung inflation and hernia reduction.

CCAM

This is a rare form of cystic lung disease. In types I and II there are multiple discernible thin-walled cysts; consideration may be given to antenatal aspiration if the cysts are large. In type III the cysts are very small and the lung appears large and hyperechoic (differentiate from bronchial obstruction and sequestration). The prognosis of this form is good in the absence of hydrops.

Bronchial cysts

These are rare.

SKELETAL DEFORMITIES

> There are over a hundred different syndromes, and it is often not possible to identify an individual one with certainty antenatally, or even occasionally postnatally (Table 1.3). Often there is no family history of skeletal problems.

Nomenclature

Bone shortening may be distal (acromelia), proximal (rhizomelia) or overall shortened (micromelia). There may be complete absence of an extremity (amelia), or there may be an absent long bone with normal hand or foot (phocomelia). Clinodactyly describes overlapping digits, polydactyly extra digits, syndactyly fused digits and arthrogryphosis contractures of the extremities.

Ultrasound approach

Measure all long bones, assessing the degree and distribution of shortening. Also look at posture (abnormal posture suggests contractures) and for evidence of subtle hand and foot anomalies (which suggest abnormalities in other systems). Are there fractures or evidence of hypomineralization (usually indicating osteogenesis imperfecta)? Is the chest circumference small (suggestive, *but not*

TABLE 1.3 Selected skeletal dysplasias

Syndrome	Epidemiology	Features
Thanatophoric dysplasia	1 : 10 000, sporadic, lethal	Severe micromelia, cloverleaf skull (14%), small chest, polyhydramnios (60%), flattened vertebral bodies, absent corpus callosum (20%)
Osteogenesis imperfecta Type I and IV	1 : 30 000, AD, usually non-lethal	Limb length normal, extremity bowing and reduced echogenicity may occur in late gestation. Different subtypes
Heterozygous achondroplasia	1 : 30 000, Spontaneous mutation or AD, usually non-lethal	Progressive rhizomelic shortening beyond 24 weeks, large skull. (If homozygous, usually at least one parent affected, lethal. Features similar to thanatophoric)
Achondrogenesis	1 : 40 000, AR, lethal	Severe micromelia, absent vertebral body ossification, poor skull ossification, occasional rib fractures, polyhydramnios
Osteogenesis imperfecta Type II	1 : 60 0000, usually sporadic, lethal	Severe micromelia with deformity, apparent thickening of limb bones, diffuse hypomineralization allowing clear visualization of the sulci. The skull may be easily compressed. Multiple rib fractures with collapse of the rib cage. Different subtypes. Differentiate from congenital hypophosphataemia (also lethal)

indicative, of lethal abnormality)? It is also important to look for extraskeletal abnormalities. The commonest dysplasias are listed in Table 1.3, but it is essential to consider a wider diagnostic list.

Clinical management

As a precise antenatal diagnosis is often difficult, it is important to involve the parents and paediatricians in decision-making about method of delivery, intrapartum monitoring, appropriateness of intrapartum caesarean section and extent of postnatal resuscitation.

NON-IMMUNE HYDROPS

There is skin oedema > 5 mm and two or more of pericardial effusion, pleural effusion, ascites (Fig. 1.16) and a large placenta in the absence of antibody to red cell antigens (compare with HDN, p. 51). The incidence is ≈ 1 : 2500 to 1 : 4000 and the mortality is 50–80%. There may be maternal problems in 80% due to polyhydramnios, pre-eclampsia or preterm labour. There may also be oligohydramnios.

There are more than 100 recognized causes, most commonly those listed below:

- cardiovascular (structural anomalies including tachyarrhythmias and CHB (30%)
- chromosomes (especially trisomies, Turner and triploidy) (15%)
- infection (10%)
- pulmonary abnormality (5%)
- renal abnormality (3%)

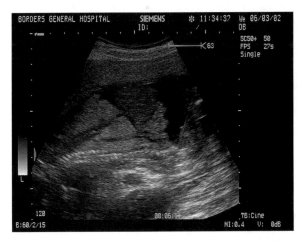

Fig. 1.16 Ascites at 20 weeks' gestation in non-immune hydrops fetalis. The lungs are to the left, with the liver and bowel surrounded by ascitic fluid.

- structural abnormalities (diaphragmatic hernia, bladder neck obstruction), blood disorders (thalassaemias, G6PD deficiency) and placental or cord lesions are rare
- the remainder are rare.

Investigation is probably best carried out in a specialist fetal medicine unit:

- Is there a history of recent infections, or a family history of congenital disorders?
- Group, antibodies and Kleihauer–Betke stain.
- FBC ± electrophoresis for haemoglobinopathies.
- Viral titres for toxoplasmosis, CMV, rubella and human parvovirus B19.
- TPHA for syphilis.
- Autoantibody screen for anti-Ro, ANF and anti-DNA.
- USS: detailed FA scan, including skeletal survey, echocardiography and Doppler.
- Amniocentesis for karyotype and culture; or FBS (only if > 22 weeks) for FBC, blood group and direct Coombs test, karyotype, viral serology and haemoglobin electrophoresis.

Management

- If there is a dysrhythmia, see page 14.
- Intrauterine transfusions of RCC may be of value in some cases, especially in parvovirus B19.
- Avoid delivery before term if possible.
- Delivery by caesarean section does not affect outcome, but allows planned paediatric care. Drainage of pleural cavities immediately prior to delivery may be helpful.
- Consider termination of pregnancy (and postmortem) if very preterm.

OTHER INHERITED CONDITIONS

α1-antitrypsin deficiency (AR)

There are more than 75 genetic variants, most of which are benign. One person in 3000 is homozygous for the PiZ gene, and about 30% will present with infantile hepatitis, which can progress to cirrhosis. A further 30% will develop early or midlife emphysema. The antenatal diagnosis of PiZ is possible using DNA from amniocentesis or CVS.

Albinism (AR but some AD or X-linked)

Incidence 1 : 20 000 LBs. There are at least 10 types.

Congenital adrenal hyperplasia (AR)

Incidence 1 : 10 000 LBs. There is usually a 21-hydroxylase deficiency, which presents with ambiguous genitalia in a female fetus or with macrogenitosomia in the male. Both sexes may present in adrenal collapse in the neonatal period. Antenatal diagnosis is possible with CVS (see also Ambiguous genitalia, p. 229).

Beckwith–Weidmann syndrome

This is characterized by a large tongue and kidneys with exomphalos (often small) and microcephaly. There are early feeding difficulties.

Cystic fibrosis (AR)

The UK gene frequency is 1 : 25 (i.e. heterozygote frequency), and an estimated overall couple risk for a live birth of around 1 : 2500. Clinically, there is respiratory, gastrointestinal, liver and pancreatic dysfunction, and azoospermia is the rule. The prognosis is very variable and although death in the age group 20–30 years still occurs, the prognosis is improving and many now live considerably longer. The health of an affected sibling is not a prognostic guide to the health of other siblings. Four mutant alleles account for 85% of the gene defects in the UK (the commonest being ∆F508), and antenatal screening for these is possible using saliva specimens, with CVS being performed if both parents are gene carriers (see also p. 200).

Cystic hygroma (MF)

Cystic hygromas probably develop from a defect in the formation of lymphatic vessels – it is likely that the lymphatic system and venous system fail to connect and lymph fluid accumulates in the jugular lymph sacs. Larger hygromas are frequently divided by septae. Check also for skin oedema, ascites, pleural and pericardial effusions, and cardiac and renal abnormalities. There is an association with aneuploidy (particularly Turner's, Down's and Edward's syndromes) and it is appropriate to offer karyotyping. If generalized hydrops is present the prognosis is bleak. Isolated hygromas may be surgically corrected postnatally and have a good prognosis. Only very rarely are they so large as to result in dystocia.

Facial clefts (MF)

Incidence 1 : 1000 LBs. These are mostly idiopathic, but are occasionally associated with rare single gene defects or chromosomal abnormalities (e.g. T13 or T18). There is also an association with benzodiazepine use, folate acid antagonists and rubella. There are other structural malformations in 15–50% of cases. Repair of unilateral or incomplete lesions gives good cosmetic results, but there is often some residual deformity with bilateral lesions. Avoid taking the baby to the SCBU if possible (to aid bonding). The risk of recurrence of isolated lesions (with normal parents) is 1 : 50 for unilateral defects and 1 : 20 for bilateral defects. Isolated cleft palate occurs in 1 : 2500 births and carries a recurrence risk of 1 : 50 for both siblings and offspring. Midline clefts are rare, and holoprosencephaly should be excluded.

Fragile X syndrome (XL)

Incidence 0.7 : 1000 male LBs, 0.4 : 1000 female LBs. This is the commonest cause of moderate mental retardation after Down's syndrome and the commonest form of inherited mental handicap. Males are usually more severely affected than females. Speech delay is common and there is an associated behavioural phenotype, with gaze aversion. The condition is caused by the expansion of a CGG triplet repeat on the X chromosome. Normal individuals have an average of 29 repeats, but for an unexplained reason this may increase to a premutation of 50–200 repeats. Those with a premutation are phenotypically normal, but the premutation is unstable during female meiosis and can expand to a full mutation of more than 200 repeats. There is an approximately 10% chance of this occurring (in the absence of a full mutation in that generation already). This causes the fragile X phenotype in 99% of males and in around 30–50% of females. Parental screening is possible and CVS may be used to identify the degree of amplification of the CGG repeats in potential offspring. (For other repeat disorders see Myotonic dystrophy and Huntington's chorea, below.)

Galactosaemia (AR)

Incidence 1 : 200 000 LBs. This transferase deficiency is usually fatal before 4 weeks of life due to cachexia and septicaemia. A lactose-free diet is essential, and recent reports have suggested that mild learning difficulties and infertility can be associated with the condition even if a strict diet is followed. Antenatal diagnosis is possible.

Haemophilia

Haemophilia A (XL) Incidence 0.2 : 1000 male LBs. There is deficiency of factor VIII. Antenatal diagnosis may be possible with specific markers or known factor VIII mutations.

Haemophilia B (XL) Incidence 0.03 : 1000 male LBs. There is deficiency of factor IX. Antenatal diagnosis may be possible.

Haemorrhagic disease of the newborn

HDN results from a lack of vitamin K (there are no enteric bacteria) and presents with systemic bleeding. The classic form occurs between days 1 and 7, although an early form occurs in infants born to mothers taking anticonvulsants, and a late (and sometimes more serious) form may also occur. Almost complete protection is given by the administration of vitamin K (1 mg IM) at the time of birth, and possibly less complete protection is provided by giving vitamin K (2 mg PO) twice in the first week (with a further oral dose at 1 month). Some epidemiological studies have found an association between IM vitamin K (as opposed to oral) and childhood leukaemias, resulting in a swing away from treatment. *Numerous large* subsequent studies have not confirmed this apparent association.

Hirschsprung's disease (MF)

Incidence 1 : 8000 LBs with a 3 : 1 male excess. If the child is male, the chance of sibling recurrence is 1 : 25. If female, this chance is 1 : 8. The risk of recurrence if one or other parent has been affected is < 1 : 100.

Huntington's chorea (AD)

Incidence 4–560 : 100 000 LBs. The onset usually occurs after the age of 30, although it may present as early as 10–15 years of age. There is dementia, mood change (usually depression) and choreoathetosis progressing to death in approximately 15 years. There is a CAG trinucleotide expansion on chromosome 4p, allowing accurate carrier and prenatal testing. (For other repeat disorders see Fragile X syndrome, above, and Myotonic dystrophy, below.)

Hurler's mucopolysaccharidosis (AR)

Incidence 1 : 40 000 LBs. This disease is fatal between 5 and 10 years of age. Antenatal diagnosis is possible.

Marfan's syndrome (AD)

Incidence 1 : 20 000 LBs. The individual is tall, doliocephalic and carries the risk of kyphoscoliosis, ectopia lentis, aortic regurgitation and dissecting aortic aneurysm. One in 10 individuals with Marfan's syndrome has a dilated aortic root and prophylactic β-blockade is recommended. Aortic-root diameter should be monitored during the pregnancy of a woman with Marfan's syndrome.

Muscular dystrophy

This refers to a group of primary muscle-wasting diseases that are genetically determined and usually progressive.

Becker muscular dystrophy (XL recessive) This is also caused by mutations (usually in-frame deletions) in the dystrophin gene. Intellectual impairment is less common and the progression is slower than with Duchenne muscular dystrophy. The two disorders can be differentiated by dystrophin analysis on muscle biopsy.

Congenital muscular dystrophy This refers to several distinct diseases, usually with AR inheritance, presenting with a floppy infant ± arthrogryphosis and contractures. The prognosis is very variable, but often good.

Duchenne muscular dystrophy (XL recessive) Incidence 0.3 : 1000 males. It is caused by mutations in the dystrophin gene. There is occasional mild intellectual impairment in 30%, and progressive muscle weakness such that the patient is usually wheelchair dependent by 10–12 years of age; 75% die before 20 years; 95% by 50 years. There may also be an associated cardiomyopathy. Two-thirds of affected boys are carriers, one-third representing new mutations. Antenatal diagnosis with CVS is possible in the 70% of families, where the dystrophin gene mutation is readily detected if the family structure is suitable for linkage analysis.

Facioscapulohumeral muscular dystrophy (often AD) There is shoulder weakness, usually coming on around 12–14 years, associated with difficulty sucking and whistling. It is usually relatively benign, but there is marked familial variation.

Limb girdle muscular dystrophy (AR) There is progressive weakness usually beginning in early adult life and often requiring a wheelchair by the age of 30.

Myotonia congenita (Thomsen's disease) (AD)

There is a non-progressive myotonia and failure to relax the grasp. Intelligence is normal.

Myotonic dystrophy (AD)

This condition characteristically presents in early or midadult life and is caused by the expansion of a CTG triplet repeat on chromosome 19. The degree of expansion correlates with severity of presentation, being largest in babies with congenital onset. There is grip and percussion myotonia with muscle weakness, particularly of proximal muscles. Other features include early cataracts and premature frontal balding. Women who have symptomatic disease are at particular risk of conceiving infants with congenital myotonic dystrophy. In this condition there is a high pregnancy loss rate, and both polyhydramnios and premature labour are common. Infants are born floppy and make little or no respiratory effort. Talipes and feeding difficulties are frequently encountered and, if the infant survives, learning difficulties and severe constipation are regular findings. A significant proportion die before 3 months of age. Antenatal diagnosis is possible using DNA from CVS or amniocentesis.

Neurofibromatosis type 1 (AD)
Incidence 1 : 2500 LBs. Café au lait patches are found on the skin and neurofibromas develop on peripheral nerve sheaths (the risk of malignancy is about 6%). The neurofibromas may be removed surgically. The condition can also be associated with phaeochromocytomas and renal artery stenosis. One in 10 gene carriers has learning difficulties.

Phenylketonuria (AR)
Incidence 1 : 15 000 LBs. There is a deficiency of the enzyme phenylalanine hydroxylase leading to a low level of tyrosine and a high, toxic level of phenylalanine. This leads to convulsions and mental retardation if untreated. Management is by giving a phenylalanine free diet. In pregnancy, the phenylalanine level should remain less than at least 500 µmol/l (but ideally 50–150 µmol/l) to minimize risks of IUGR, mental retardation and CHD (especially Fallot's tetralogy). There should also be tyrosine supplementation (aiming to maintain the tyrosine level at 60–90 µmol/l).

Radiation
Fetal doses resulting from most conventional diagnostic procedures have no increased association with fetal death, malformation or the impairment of fetal development. The threshold dose above which there are risks of gross malformation or fetal demise is 250–500 mGy at < 8 weeks' gestation. After 8 weeks, gross malformations are only rarely seen, but the threshold for demise up to 20 weeks is > 500 mGy, and from then until term it is > 1000 mGy. The risk of radiation-induced genetic disease in descendants of the unborn child is unknown, but there are no human data to suggest a risk, and there is no indication for TOP or the use of invasive investigations (e.g. amniocentesis).

The lifetime risk of inducing cancer after fetal exposure to 25-mGy is 0.5%. A CXR exposes the fetus to < 0.01 mGy, a pelvis view to 1.1 mGy, an IVU to 1.7 mGy, a ^{99m}Tc lung scan to 0.2 mGy, a CT of the head to < 0.005 mGy, and a pelvic CT to 25 mGy (although the exposure from CT pelvimetry is only 0.2 mGy) (National Radiological Protection Board 2004).

Tay–Sachs disease (AR)

The gene frequency is 1 : 30 in Ashkenazi Jews, but is rare in other groups. There is a build up of gangliosides within the CNS leading to retardation, paralysis and blindness. By the age of 4 years, the child is usually dead or in a vegetative state. Carriers may be screened by measuring the level of hexosaminidase A in leukocytes.

Teratomas (MF)

These are usually sacrococcygeal and are treatable in early neonatal life with surgery. Hydrops may develop in the second trimester secondary to arteriovenous shunting. However, 10–30% are malignant and, although these are indistinguishable from the benign form on USS, the prognosis following chemotherapy is good. Delivery is usually by caesarean section on account of the size of the tumour. There are numerous other rare soft-tissue cysts or tumours which may occur at different sites.

Tuberous sclerosis (AD)

Incidence 1 : 50 000 LBs. There are gliomas, which only very rarely become malignant. The clinical presentation is with infantile spasms and mental retardation from birth. In 30% of cases there are also rhabdomyomas. Antenatal diagnosis with CVS or amniocentesis may be possible.

Umbilical artery (MF)

A single umbilical artery is associated with other abnormalities in around 20% of fetuses, particularly of the urinary tract, heart and gastrointestinal system. There is an association with aneuploidy and a 10–20% association with IUGR.

Von Willebrand disease (AD)

This is due to a deficiency of factor VIII carrier protein and manifests as platelet disorder (e.g. bleeding after surgery). Diagnosis is made by demonstrating reduced platelet aggregation with ristocetin. Antenatal diagnosis is possible.

VATER association

This refers to a condition in which there are vertebral, anal, tracheal, esophageal and renal lesions. (Also, extended to VACTERL by adding cardiac and limb abnormalities.) It may result from abnormal expression of an embryonic gene involved in the development of multiple systems.

DRUGS IN PREGNANCY

The statement that all drugs are potential teratogens may seem harsh, but it emphasizes that one can never confirm the safety of any drug in pregnancy; one can only report on problems that seem to have arisen. As a general principle, all drugs should be avoided in pregnancy unless clinical benefits are likely to outweigh the risks to the fetus. A useful treatment, however, should not be stopped without good reason.

The major body structures are formed in about the first 12 weeks or so and drug treatment before this time may cause a teratogenic effect. If a drug is given after this time it will not produce a major anatomical defect, but may affect the growth and development of the baby.

See Table 1.4 and The British National Formulary Appendices 4 and 5 (new editions 6 monthly).

TABLE 1.4 Drugs in pregnancy

Class of Drug	Drug	Risk to fetus
Local anaesthetics	Prilocaine	Methaemoglobinaemia may occur if used in epidural infusions. Use lidocaine (lignocaine) or bupivacaine instead
General anaesthetics	All agents	Any risks are probably related to large doses of barbiturates for induction and to the possible teratogenic risks of hypoxia itself. There is some animal evidence to suggest an increased risk of miscarriage after exposure to anaesthetic gases, although there is no evidence that the miscarriage rate is greater in exposed theatre personnel
Analgesics	Aspirin	There were no significant problems associated with low dose aspirin use in the CLASP report (Lancet 1994;343:619).

(Continued)

TABLE 1.4 Drugs in pregnancy (Continued)

Class of Drug	Drug	Risk to fetus
		Analgesic doses may lead to impaired platelet function and an increased risk of haemorrhage
	Indometacin and other PG inhibitors	Cause impairment of renal function and may lead to premature closure of the ductus arteriosis. There may also be an association with persistent pulmonary hypertension in the newborn
	Opiates/opioids	See p. 171
	Paracetamol	Thought to be safe for use in pregnancy
Antacids and ulcer healing drugs	Alkalis	Thought to be safe for use in pregnancy
	Cimetidine	Avoid as may have anti-androgenic effects
	Omeprazole	Toxicity in animal studies. Avoid
	Ranitidine	No known problems
Antiarrhythmics	Amiodarone	Theoretical risk of depressing fetal thyroid. Avoid
Antibiotics	Aminoglycosides	There is a risk of fetal ototoxicity. Monitor levels
	Chloramphenicol	The risk of 'grey baby syndrome' from use around term is small
	Co-trimoxazole	The sulfa component may displace bilirubin and cause kernicterus. There is also some evidence of teratogenesis (trimethoprim is a folate antagonist). Both components should be avoided in pregnancy

(Continued)

TABLE 1.4 Drugs in pregnancy (Continued)

Class of Drug	Drug	Risk to fetus
	Erythromycin	Thought to be safe for use in pregnancy
	Fluconazole	Toxicity at high doses in animal studies – avoid use in pregnancy
	Fluoroquinolones (e.g. ciprofloxacin)	These cause arthropathy in animal studies. Norfloxacin has also been shown to be embryocidal in animal studies. Avoid
	Metronidazole	There is growing evidence to support its safety in pregnancy
	Penicillins	Thought to be safe for use in pregnancy
	Tetracyclines	Are contraindicated in pregnancy as they become permanently incorporated into growing bones and deciduous teeth leading to discolouration. It affects skeletal development in animal studies only. Avoid
Anticoagulants	Warfarin and heparin	See page 206
Anticonvulsants (see also p. 174)	Carbamazepine	There is a risk of craniofacial defects, neural tube defects, and developmental delay. There is also a risk of neonatal haemorrhage – give maternal vitamin K in late pregnancy and neonatal vitamin K at birth
	Gabapentin, lamotrigine and vigabatrin	Growing evidence to support safety of lamotrigine. There are significant concerns about vigabatrin and gabapentin
	Phenobarbital	There may be teratogenic problems.

(Continued)

TABLE 1.4 Drugs in pregnancy (Continued)

Class of Drug	Drug	Risk to fetus
		There is a risk of neonatal haemorrhage – give maternal vitamin K in late pregnancy and neonatal vitamin K at birth (p. 33)
	Phenytoin	There are significant teratogenic concerns, particularly with cardiac abnormalities, mental retardation, craniofacial defects and diaphragmatic herniae. Serum folate levels may be lowered, so maternal folate supplements are warranted. There is also a risk of neonatal haemorrhage – give maternal vitamin K in late pregnancy and neonatal vitamin K at birth (p. 33)
	Primadone	As for phenytoin
	Sodium valproate	There is an increase in the incidence of neural tube defects, microcephaly and cardiac abnormalities. Give folic acid preconceptually or as soon as possible in the first trimester (p. 17)
Antidepressants	MAOIs	Very limited data suggests risk of malformations. Avoid in all stages of pregnancy
	Lithium	Exposure in the first trimester has been linked with congenital heart disease. Neonatal goitre, hypotonia, cyanosis, lethargy and cardiac arrhythmias have resulted from later transplacental exposure. Avoid if possible but, if used, monitor serum levels closely

(Continued)

TABLE 1.4 Drugs in pregnancy (Continued)

Class of Drug	Drug	Risk to fetus
	SSRIs	Growing evidence to support the safety of fluoxetine
	Tricyclic antidepressants	Relatively safe in pregnancy
Anti-hypertensives	ACE inhibitors	May adversely affect fetal BP and renal function in fetus and newborn. Also possible skull defects. Avoid
	Methyl-dopa	This is widely used and is thought to be safe although there are reports of ileus with very high doses. There may be a false positive Coombs test in the fetus
	β-Blockers	Possible association with IUGR, and more definite associations with neonatal bradycardia and neonatal hypoglycaemia
	Prochlorperazine	Thought to be safe for use in pregnancy
Antihistamines	Chlorphenamine (chlorpheniramine), terfenadine	Chlorphenamine is thought to be safe in pregnancy. There is little experience with the newer preparations
Antimalarials	All preparations	For prophylaxis, chloroquine is preferred. In treatment of malarial infection, benefits far outweigh the risks
Antimitotics	Idoxuridine	There is evidence of animal teratogenesis. Avoid
	Podophyllin	There are reports of teratogenesis and fetal death after topical wart treatment. Avoid

(Continued)

TABLE 1.4 Drugs in pregnancy (Continued)

Class of Drug	Drug	Risk to fetus
Antipsychotic drugs	Chlorpromazine and related phenothiazines	No consistent teratogenic effect has been demonstrated. If antipsychotic drugs are required, chlorpromazine and trifluoperazine are probably the ones of choice. Extrapyramidal effects are occasionally seen in the neonate. There is a relatively higher incidence of problems with depot preparations
	Haloperidol	There are several poorly documented reports of limb reduction deformities. Extrapyramidal reactions in the newborn have been described
Antithyroid drugs	Carbimazole, propylthiouracil	Can be used if indicated (see p. 207)
Antivirals	Aciclovir	Experience small. There is only limited absorption from topical preparations
Bronchodilators	Inhaled preparations	All inhaled preparations, including inhaled steroids, are considered safe in pregnancy
Diuretics	Thiazides	First trimester exposure may cause an increased risk of congenital defects. Neonatal thrombocytopenia and hypoglycaemia may occur if used near term. Avoid
	Furosemide (frusemide)	May lead to reduced placental perfusion. Avoid
Hypoglycaemics	Chlorpropramide, tolbutamide	May cause neonatal hypoglycaemia
Iron supplements	Many preparations	Are thought to be safe

(Continued)

TABLE 1.4 Drugs in pregnancy (Continued)

Class of Drug	Drug	Risk to fetus
Retinoids	Etretinate, isotretinoin	High risk of fetal malformation sufficient to consider TOP. Contraception should be used from 1 month before to at least 2 years after stopping treatment. Also avoid topical treatment
Sedatives/ tranquillizers	Benzodiazepines	See page 171
Sex hormones	Androgens (including danazol)	Small risk of causing masculinization of a female fetus. Avoid
	Oestrogens	May cause urogenital defects in a male fetus. Stilboestrol is associated with later vaginal adenocarcinoma. Avoid
	Progestogens	May cause masculinization of a female fetus. Avoid
	Combined oral contraceptive	Meta-analysis does not support any evidence of teratogenesis
Steroids		Although there are associations with fetal abnormality in animal studies, particularly cleft palate, there have been no teratogenic effects demonstrated in humans despite extensive usage. Fetal adrenal suppression possible with > 10 mg prednisolone/day
Vaccines		There is a theoretical risk of teratogenic problems from vaccines. On principle only, live vaccines (BCG, MMR, oral polio vaccine, oral typhoid, yellow fever) should be avoided if possible. Nonetheless, for any vaccine, the protective

(Continued)

TABLE 1.4 Drugs in pregnancy (Continued)		
Class of Drug	Drug	Risk to fetus
		benefits probably outweigh any potential risks
Vitamin	A	Excessive doses in the first trimester may be teratogenic
	D	There may be a risk of skeletal abnormalities in high dose regimens.

CHAPTER 2

ANTENATAL PROBLEMS

BREECH PRESENTATION

> The incidence of breech presentation is 40% at 20 weeks, 25% at 32 weeks and 3% at term, with the chance of spontaneous version after 38 weeks less than 4%. It is associated with multiple pregnancy, bicornuate uterus, fibroids, placenta praevia, polyhydramnios and oligohydramnios. At term, 65% of breech presentations are frank (extended). The remainder are flexed or footling (the latter carries a 5–20% risk of cord prolapse).

Planned caesarean section is associated with less perinatal mortality and serious neonatal morbidity than planned vaginal birth for the term fetus in the breech presentation; serious maternal complications are similar between the groups (Lancet 2000;1375:356).

OPTIONS

External cephalic version

All women with an uncomplicated breech pregnancy at term (37–42 weeks) should be offered ECV at around 38 weeks' gestation. ECV is contraindicated with placenta praevia, multiple pregnancy, APH and relatively contraindicated in those with pre-eclampsia, IUGR and a previous caesarean section. Check a CTG and ultrasound. Some obstetricians like the patient to be fasted and prepared for theatre. Although this is almost never necessary, it is reasonable to have access to theatre close at hand. It is most likely to be successful when the presenting part is free, the head is easy to palpate and the uterus feels soft.

Establish a ritodrine IVI at 200 µg/min for 15 minutes (see p. 95). Ask the mother to lie flat with a 30° lateral tilt. Scanning gel allows easier manipulation and permits scanning during the procedure if required. Disengage the breech with the scan probe or hands, and then attempt to rotate in the direction the baby is facing (i.e. forward role/somersault). Check the FH every 2 minutes. If unsuccessful return to breech rather than leave transverse. Give anti-D 500 IU IM if rhesus negative. Success rate of version ≈ 30% for primigravidae and ≈ 60% for parous women.

Caesarean section

The Lancet trial quoted above considers term pregnancies only. Nonetheless, it is probably also advisable to carry out a caesarean section in preterm deliveries as there is the additional risk of the cervix closing around the neck after delivery of the breech. Whether caesarean section is also appropriate in extreme prematurity is more difficult to assess as operative delivery may be traumatic (a De Lees or classic incision may help).

Vaginal delivery (for delivery technique, see p. 111)

This may occasionally be considered appropriate by some clinicians if the estimated fetal weight is < 3.8 kg with no fetal compromise, pre-eclampsia or placenta praevia. Ideally the onset of labour should be spontaneous, the breech frank or flexed (but not footling) and the liquor volume normal. The risks include intracranial injury, widespread bruising, damage to internal organs, spinal cord transection, umbilical cord prolapse and hypoxia following obstruction of the after-coming head (the incidence of intrapartum caesarean section in those planning a vaginal breech delivery in the UK is approximately 30–50%). Those not assessed antenatally and presenting in advanced labour with an engaged breech usually deliver without adverse consequences.

FETAL MONITORING

> **Antenatal monitoring is used in the hope of identifying fetal compromise in utero. Resist the temptation to act on one abnormality when all else seems normal if the risks to the fetus of an early delivery are high. It is always essential to assess the complete clinical picture when considering the results of investigations, particularly the previous obstetric history, medical history, fetal growth, movements and other investigations.**

Fetal movements

These can be used as a screening test for further investigations. The patient is often asked to choose a starting time (usually 9 a.m.) and record how long it takes to feel 10 separate movements. If there have been < 10 movements by, say, 5 p.m. she is asked to contact for further tests (e.g. CTG). There is great variation in what may be considered as normal, and 'a change in the usual movements' may be

TABLE 2.1 Parameters of the biophysical profile	
CTG	More than 2 accelerations of 15 bpm lasting longer than 15 seconds in 20 minutes
Fetal breathing	Lasting more than 30 seconds in 30 minutes
Fetal movements	More than 3 limb or trunk movements in 30 minutes
Fetal tone	One return to flexion (of neck) after extension, or one hand opening and closing
Liquor	More than 3 cm depth in 2 planes

Biophysical profile

Five parameters are assessed, scored as 2 each, and the total out of 10 used to give an indication of fetal well-being (Table 2.1). Of all the parameters, liquor volume is probably the most predictive of fetal well-being. The CTG may be considered separately (and the score therefore given out of 8). Although available for many years the score is time consuming and there is little evidence of benefit over the non-stress CTG or Doppler. There is inadequate evidence to substantiate the usefulness of this technique.

Overall interpretation

Figure 2.2 illustrates the probable sequence of events in fetal decompensation. As umbilical Doppler abnormalities are the first to appear, it is logical to use Doppler as the main screening tool. Thereafter, the optimal surveillance strategy in fetuses with absent or reduced end-diastolic flow is unclear but some form of frequent (e.g. daily) monitoring with CTGs, biophysical profile and further Doppler studies seems appropriate. The timing of the delivery will be decided by weighing up the risks of leaving the baby in utero against the risks of prematurity, but delivery is likely to be appropriate when the CTG becomes pathological (decelerations or reduced variability), the biophysical profile becomes abnormal (e.g. < 4) or there is reversal of end-diastolic flow. If IUGR is suspected before 34–36 weeks, it is appropriate to consider giving steroids to the mother to enhance fetal lung maturation.

The actual mode of delivery depends on the individual circumstances, but it must be remembered that the placental reserve of some of these fetuses may be low and careful monitoring in labour is required. Early recourse to caesarean section is appropriate if the monitoring shows signs of fetal compromise. Prelabour caesarean section may be appropriate if there are major prelabour concerns about fetal well-being.

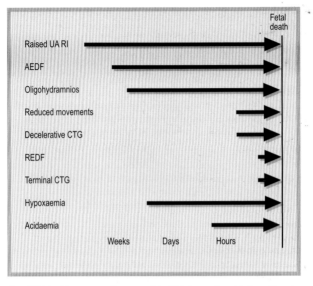

Fig. 2.2 The 'decompensation cascade' of fetal growth restriction. Absent end-diastolic flow (AEDF) is a relatively early sign of hypoxaemia, with reduced fetal movements, cardiotocographic abnormalities and reversed end-diastolic flow (REDF) late features. UA RI: uterine artery resistance index. (Adapted from Drife J, Magowan B. Clinical Obstetrics and Gynaecology, Saunders 2004, with permission.)

HAEMOLYTIC DISEASE OF THE NEWBORN

Maternal IgG antibodies to fetal red cell antigens cross the placenta and cause fetal haemolysis, anaemia and hydrops fetalis. Initial sensitization usually occurs at delivery, but may also occur with PV bleeding at any stage, amniocentesis, ECV or at some unrecognized event (10% of affected pregnancies). It tends to become more severe with subsequent pregnancies: if the last baby died from rhesus haemolytic disease the chance of successful outcome in the next pregnancy is < 50%. There are > 700 known antigens, but rhesus accounts for more than 95% of haemolytic disease.

PROPHYLAXIS

Prophylaxis is only available for the 'D' antigen. It is available in 250, 500, 2500 and 5000 IU/vial. A dose of 125 IU is sufficient to react with 1–2 ml of fetal blood.

Antenatal

Anti-D should be given to Rhesus-negative mothers following any PV bleeding in pregnancy (including ectopic, miscarriage, termination, CVS, amniocentesis, cordocentesis, ECV, external trauma and APH).

- If < 20 weeks, give 250 IU IM stat.
- If > 20 weeks, give an initial 500 IU IM stat. and carry out a Kleihauer test (estimates the volume of fetal blood transfused). Give more anti-D if indicated by the Kleihauer result.
- If there is ongoing intermittent bleeding, repeat the anti-D 6-weekly.

Prophylaxis is likely to be more effective if anti-D is given to all Rhesus-negative mothers routinely in the third trimester (either 500 IU at 28 and 34 weeks, or a single larger dose early in the third trimester).

Postnatal

If the mother is Rhesus negative and the baby Rhesus positive, check a Kleihauer test and give an initial 500 IU anti-D IM stat. More anti-D may be required following the Kleihauer result. The anti-D should be administered within 72 hours.

SCREENING

Approximately 15% of women in the UK are Rhesus negative. All women should be screened for all antibodies at booking. The maternal serum level of the antibody (usually anti-D) is used as an initial screening test for further action. There are regional variations, but an example of when to check levels is shown in Table 2.2.

RHESUS DISEASE

Without recourse to prophylaxis, 1% of Rhesus-negative mothers would develop anti-D in their first pregnancy and 3–5% in subsequent pregnancies. If antibody is detected, check the paternal genotype. If the father is homozygous for 'd', then both he and the fetus will be Rhesus negative, making significant Rhesus disease unlikely. If

TABLE 2.2 Potential screening programme for antibodies in haemolytic disease of the newborn

All pregnant women (including RhD +ve)	ABO + RhD group and antibody screen	At 10–16 weeks
	RhD group and antibody screen	At 28–36 weeks
Patients with auto-antibodies Anti-D, C or Kell related	Antibody screen/titre	At least monthly to 28 weeks then 2 weekly to term
Other antibodies	Antibody screen/titre	At 28–36 weeks, thereafter on titre

heterozygous for 'D', there is a 50% chance that the fetus will be Rhesus positive and, if homozygous, the chance is 100%. Those mothers with rising antibody levels are sometimes assessed by amniocentesis as outlined below. It is probably more appropriate, however, to refer them to a specialist fetal medicine unit for fetal blood sampling. If the previous pregnancy has been complicated by Rhesus iso-immunization, perform the first invasive investigation 10 weeks before the previous intrauterine death, intrauterine transfusion or delivery. Also consider investigations with a rising level of maternal antibody level, or if there are reduced fetal movements, or if there is ultrasound evidence of fetal anaemia (e.g. ascites, cardiomegaly, pleural effusions or polyhydramnios). Severe disease is rare if the maternal antibody is < 4 IU/ml. The risk of severe disease is moderate if maternal antibody is 4–15 IU/ml, and there is a risk of severe anaemia in 50% of fetuses when the level is > 15 IU/ml. There is now an established role to use fetal middle cerebral artery Doppler flow studies to screen for moderate or severe anaemia (Fig. 2.3). Such anaemia is unlikely with normal Doppler studies (N Eng J Med 2000;342:9–14).

Amniocentesis

This is carried out to measure amniotic fluid bilirubin levels with spectrophotometry at OD_{450} (note that artefactual levels occur following chronic maternal steroid administration). The result is plotted on a Liley chart to decide between conservative management, intrauterine transfusion or delivery. There is evidence, however, that serum levels of anti-D correlate so well with amniocentesis findings that amniocentesis is not necessary, fetal blood sampling being preferable.

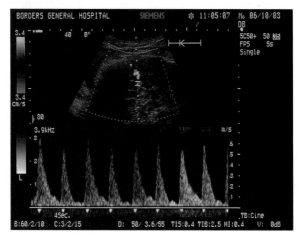

Fig. 2.3 In fetuses without hydrops who are at risk of maternal red-cell isoimmunization, moderate and severe anaemia can be detected by Doppler studies of the middle cerebral artery.

Fetal blood sampling

This is carried out under ultrasound guidance. The blood group can be checked and if the haematocrit (or in some centres haemoglobin) is low the fetus is transfused with a calculated volume of group O Rhesus-negative blood which has been cross-matched to the mother's own serum. The transfusion may be given intraperitoneally or by the intravascular route. Fetal blood sampling carries the risk of cord haematoma, bradycardia, intrauterine death and further sensitization of the mother to fetal red cell antigens. It is usually repeated again every 2 weeks and delivery performed around 36 weeks.

OTHER ANTIBODIES

Other antigens

Many of these (e.g. anti-c, Kell, e, Ce, Fy^a, Jk^a, C^w) are poorly developed on the red cell surface and usually stimulate only low levels of antibody production, often of the IgM category (which does not cross the placenta). Some will, however, cause significant HDN. Note particularly that anti-Kell causes marrow aplasia rather than HDN, and that serum antibody levels and the OD$_{450}$ are poor predictors of disease severity. It is important to check the paternal genotype to assess the risk of anti-Kell disease and FBS must be used to assess disease severity. The inheritance is AD, the gene being called K (most people are 'k' positive, also termed 'cellano' positive). Anti-Le^a, Le^b, Lu^a, P, N, Xg^a and Kn^a have not been associated with HDN.

Du antigen

Treat as Rhesus negative for the purposes of haemolytic disease of the newborn.

ABO

In 15% of pregnancies the mother will be group O and the fetus A or B. This rarely causes significant HDN and the risk to the fetus is very low. The severity in subsequent pregnancies is unpredictable owing to the variability of red cell protein expression. ABO incompatibility in Rhesus-negative mothers very much reduces the likelihood of Rhesus iso-immunization to a Rhesus-positive fetus. No antenatal investigations are warranted.

HYPEREMESIS GRAVIDARUM

> **Nausea and vomiting occur in 50–80% of pregnancies in the first trimester. Inability to keep down fluids or solids leads to weight loss (2 to > 5 kg), dehydration and electrolyte disturbances. Only very rarely does it lead to vitamin B deficiency (polyneuropathy), liver failure, renal failure and fetal or maternal death.**

Check

- U&E, haematocrit, MSU, urine for ketones and TFTs (see Hyperthyroidism, p. 208).
- LFTs if severe or prolonged (↓albumin, ↑transaminases, PTR normal).
- USS: ? multiple pregnancy or trophoblastic disease.
- Social aspects of admission.

Treatment

Admission and IV fluids are usually sufficient by themselves to reduce nausea and should be the only initial management. The patient should eat a little often. Antiemetics should be used only if the vomiting is not settling. The risk of teratogenesis with these antiemetics is considered to be low:

- metoclopramide 10 mg IM/IV TID
- cyclizine 50 g IM/IV TID
- prochlorperazine 12.5 g IM TID
- chlorpromazine 100 mg suppository QID (may lead to jaundice and extrapyramidal side-effects in the fetus).

If the vomiting is prolonged, severe and unresponsive to standard management there are some data to suggest that prednisolone 20 mg PO BD or TID or ondansetron 8 mg PO BD or 16 mg/day PR may be of help. Also consider enteral feeding (or TPN) and vitamin B supplementation if very severe. Abnormal LFTs respond rapidly to correction of dehydration and malnutrition.

EATING DISORDERS

The incidence of bulimia and anorexia nervosa in pregnancy is less than in the non-pregnant population.

Bulimia
Those with bulimia tend to improve in later pregnancy and often become worse again after delivery. There may be a slightly greater incidence of fetal anomaly.

Anorexia nervosa
Those with anorexia may become worse as pregnancy advances. The incidence of low-birth-weight infants is increased, particularly if ovulation induction has been used to assist conception. The perinatal mortality is also greater. Delay ovulation induction until the weight is > 45 kg.

INTRAUTERINE DEATH

This is defined as intrauterine death after 24 weeks' gestation. If managed conservatively, 80% will labour within 2 weeks and 90% within 3 weeks. The risk of maternal coagulopathy is rare before 3–4 weeks has elapsed from the time of the IUD (with the exception of abruption).

Causes

- Fetal causes: anomaly (including chromosomal), immune and non-immune hydrops fetalis, abruption and cord accidents.
- Maternal causes: pre-eclampsia and other medical disorders (renal, diabetes mellitus, infection, connective tissue disorders, impaired placental function).
- In at least 20% of cases no cause is found.

Check

- FBC and clotting.
- Kleihauer–Betke stain (? feto-maternal transfusion).
- HbA1C and random glucose.
- Lupus anticoagulant, anticardiolipin antibodies and thrombophilia screen (associated with impaired fetal outcome, see p. 161).
- Toxoplasma. Rubella, CMV and parvovirus B_{19} antibodies (looking for the presence of IgM, or a change in IgG from the booking sample).

If clinically there has been an abruption, see page 106. Otherwise induce labour, ideally with mifepristone and misoprostol, but avoid membrane rupture until as late as possible as there is a high chance of chorioamnionitis.

After-care

- Counselling.
- Offer of both religious support and time alone with the baby is essential.
- Also offer photos, handprints, a hair lock and help with the funeral arrangements.
- Discuss postmortem and chromosome studies.
- The parents are required to take a Stillbirth Certificate to the Registrar of Births and Deaths within 42 days.
- Discuss any local support group (e.g. SANDS).
- Arrange contraception if required.
- Arrange a follow-up appointment (in about 6 weeks) to discuss the results.

MINOR DISORDERS OF PREGNANCY

Anaemia

As there is a physiological fall in haemoglobin as pregnancy advances, there is controversy about the treatment of mild anaemia (e.g. Hb 8–10 g/dl). Iron supplements may lead to GI side-effects, have no proven benefits and carry theoretical worries about increasing the risks of 'sludging' within the placenta. On the other hand, iron supplements have no proven harmful effects, and may lead to improvements in mitochondrial function and generalized well-being. Most practitioners will prescribe oral $FeSO_4$ if the Hb is < 10 g/dl or if the MCV is low (e.g. < 80 fl). If MCV very low, consider haemoglobinopathy (? electrophoresis). Oral iron is very well absorbed and the only indication for parenteral iron is when there are compliance worries or prohibitive side-effects with the oral route. Parenteral iron should never be given in thalassaemia.

Backache
This occurs as ligaments relax. A support brace may help.

Carpal tunnel syndrome
The median nerve, which supplies the thumb, index and middle fingers, is compressed under the flexor retinaculum. Holding the wrist hyperflexed for 2 minutes reproduces the symptoms (this is more accurate than Tinel's test). Treatment is with splints, a local hydrocortisone injection or division of the retinaculum.

Constipation
This is common and usually responds to a high-fibre diet or laxatives. Avoid stimulant laxatives.

Cramps in the legs
This affects around a third of women in pregnancy and will be severe in 5%. There is no useful treatment and quinine should not be used.

Itching
This may be localized to the perineum or may be generalized. Localized itching may be due to infection (particularly candidiasis but, less commonly, pediculosis pubis or trichomonas vaginalis). Generalized itching may occur with eczema, urticaria or scabies. If there is a systemic rash, consider one of the four pregnancy-associated dermatoses (Table 2.3). Itching may also be due to intrahepatic cholestasis of pregnancy (see p. 177).

Nausea
See Hyperemesis, p. 55.

TABLE 2.3 Dermatoses of pregnancy

	Incidence	Features	Usual timing of onset	Fetal problems	Treatment
Pemphigoid gestationis	1 : 10 000	Pruritic erythematous papules, plaques and wheals spreading from the peri-umbilical area to the breasts, thighs and palms. Diagnosed by the presence of immunofluorescence of biopsy	9 weeks' gestation to 7 weeks' postpartum	IUGR and increased fetal abnormality	Antihistamines, topical steroids, systemic steroids and rarely plasmapheresis
Polymorphic eruption of pregnancy	1 : 240	Urticaria and vesicles (with no bullae), rarely occurring in the peri-umbilical area	32 weeks' gestation to term	None	Antihistamines and topical steroids
Prurigo of pregnancy	1 : 300	Excoriated pustules on extensor surfaces	25–30 weeks' gestation	None	Antihistamines and topical steroids
Pruritic folliculitis		Acneiform rash	16–40 weeks' gestation	None	Topical steroids

Oedema

This is very common in the ankle. Exclude pre-eclampsia and consider DVT. Elevation and support stockings are a help. Diuretics should not be used.

Reflux oesophagitis and heartburn

These occur secondary to relaxation of the oesophageal sphincter and pressure from the gravid uterus. Small meals should be taken often and cigarettes avoided. Antacids are helpful and there has been no reported teratogenicity with ranitidine.

Urinary frequency and stress incontinence

These usually resolve postnatally, but pelvic floor exercises can be commenced antenatally. Exclude a UTI.

MULTIPLE PREGNANCY

> **The UK incidence of twins is 12 : 1000 (3 : 1000 of these are monozygous). Worldwide the incidence ranges from 54 : 1000 in Nigeria to 4 : 1000 in Japan with the differences being almost entirely due to variations in dizygous rates. The incidence is higher with ovulation induction (e.g. with clomifene 10%, with gonadotrophins 30%). The perinatal mortality in twin pregnancies is four or five times higher than for singleton pregnancies, largely related to preterm delivery (40% deliver before 37 weeks compared with 6% in singletons), IUGR, feto-fetal transfusion sequence (FFTS), malpresentation and an increased incidence of congenital malformations (monozygotic only).**

Chorionicity (i.e. number of placentae)

All dizygous pregnancies are dichorionic, and therefore have separate chorions and amnions. The placental tissue may appear to be continuous, but there are no significant vascular communications between the fetuses. Monozygotic pregnancies may also be dichorionic, but may be monochorionic diamniotic or monochorionic monoamniotic (Fig. 2.4). Most monochorionic placentas have interfetal vascular connections (Table 2.4).

Chorionicity determination is essential to allow risk stratification (Table 2.5), and has key implications for prenatal diagnosis and antenatal monitoring. It is most easily determined in the first or early second trimester:

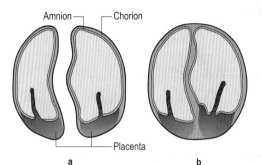

Amnion — Chorion

Placenta

a　　　　　b

c　　　　　d

Fig. 2.4 Chorionicity in monozygotic pregnancies. (Adapted from Drife J, Magowan B. Clinical Obstetrics and Gynaecology, Saunders 2004, with permission.)

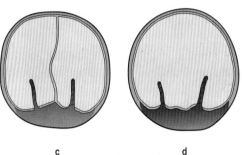

TABLE 2.4 Chorionicity			
Chorionicity	Incidence (%)		Timing of separation (days)
Dichorionic	Diamniotic	30	Separation < 4
Monochorionic	Diamniotic	66	Separation 4–7
Monochorionic	Monoamniotic	3	Separation 7–14
Conjoined		< 1	Separation > 14

- Widely separated first trimester sacs or separate placentae are dichorionic.
- Those with a 'lambda' or 'twin-peak' sign at the membrane insertion are dichorionic.
- Those with a dividing membrane > 2 mm are often dichorionic.
- Different sex fetuses are always dichorionic (and dizygous).

TABLE 2.5 Chorionicity and pregnancy outcome		
	Dichorionic (%)	Monochorionic (%)
Fetal loss before 24 weeks	1.8	12.2
Fetal loss after 24 weeks	1.6	2.8
Delivery before 32 weeks	5.5	9.2

The high early fetal mortality in monochorionic pregnancy before 24 weeks is probably largely due to severe early onset FFTS.

Fetal abnormality
The incidence is no different per fetus in a dichorionic pregnancy compared to a singleton pregnancy, but the incidence of fetal abnormality is greater with monochorionicity (especially hydrocephalus, GI atresia and cardiac defects).

Structural defects These are usually confined to one twin (i.e. non-concordant), e.g. if there is an NTD in one twin, the other twin is normal in > 90%. All multiple pregnancies should be offered a detailed midtrimester USS. Selective termination with intracardiac KCl is possible in dichorionic pregnancies only, and is most safely carried out before 16–20 weeks.

Chromosomal abnormalities These are often discordant in dizygotic twins and almost always concordant in monozygotic twins. NT measurement is more appropriate than serum screening for multiple pregnancies (but note that NT may be slightly increased in normal monochorionic gestations). Two amniocenteses are required in dichorionic pregnancies (great care must be taken to document which sample has come from which sac). CVS is not appropriate for twin pregnancies as it is difficult to be sure that both placentas have been sampled, particularly if they are lying close together.

Management of pregnancy
At the initial visit:

- A small proportion of twins diagnosed in the first trimester will proceed only as singletons despite the absence of PV loss. Parents should be told this if twins are diagnosed in the first trimester. Ensure chorionicity is established at the first scan. Consider starting FeSO$_4$ 200 mg/day and folate 5 mg/day.
- The parents are often quite surprised initially, so focus on the positive aspects while outlining that closer monitoring will be

required. A further visit at least a few days later is appropriate for more detail, including a full discussion about whether antenatal screening should be performed, opening up to them at that stage the potential problems of finding one normal and one abnormal twin.

Thereafter, scan at:

- 18 weeks for growth discrepancy ± fetal abnormality if the patient wishes
- 22 weeks and 2 weekly thereafter for monochorionic pregnancies
- 24 weeks and 3–4 weekly thereafter for dichorionic pregnancies.

Doppler, CTG and biophysical profile studies can be used if appropriate.

Antenatal problems specific to multiple pregnancies

Feto-fetal transfusion sequence (FFTS) (Twin–twin transfusion syndrome). This complicates 4–35% of monochorionic multiple pregnancies and accounts for ≈ 15% of perinatal mortality in twins. The recipient develops polyhydramnios with raised amniotic pressure, while the donor develops oliguria, oligohydramnios and growth restriction. This amniotic fluid discordancy is used to establish the diagnosis and is supported by discordant growth measurements. Contrary to previous thinking, the haemoglobin levels are often not discordant. There are two main treatment options in addition to delivery with evidence to suggest that serial amniodrainage is most appropriate in milder forms, and laser surgery for the more severe.

- *Serial amniodrainage.* This consists of performing amniocentesis (inserting a needle into the gestational sac), once or as frequently as required, to eliminate excessive fluid. The average survival achieved by amniodrainage is about 65%, but neurodevelopmental impairment has been described to be around 20% of surviving infants.
- *Fetoscopic laser surgery.* This is a more specialized treatment. Direct vision of the placenta is achieved through an endoscope, and the communicating vessels are identified and destroyed with a laser. The survival rate is probably over 80%, with neurological damage in surviving infants around 5% at 1 year of age. Three randomized trials are ongoing at the time of writing, with recruitment for the *www.eurofetus.org* trial complete.

Twins with one fetal death First-trimester IUD in a twin has not been shown to have adverse consequences for the survivor. This probably also holds true for the early second trimester, but loss in the late second or third trimester commonly precipitates labour and a high proportion will have delivered within a few weeks. Prognosis for a surviving dichorionic fetus is then influenced primarily by its gestation. When a monochorionic twin dies in utero, however, there are additional risks of death (approximately 20%) or cerebral damage (approximately 25%) in the co-twin. It is unlikely that immediate delivery will affect the risk of cerebral injury in the survivor.

Twin reversed arterial perfusion sequence (acardia) This is very rare and there is a high incidence of mortality in the donor twin due to intrauterine cardiac failure and prematurity. Cord ligation has been used in some cases.

The commonest twin presentations are cephalic/cephalic (40%), cephalic/ breech (40%), breech/cephalic (10%) and others, e.g. transverse (10%). Triplets and higher order multiples are probably best delivered by caesarean section. In general with twins, providing the first twin is cephalic and there are no complications, vaginal delivery is probably appropriate. With significant growth discordance, particularly if the second twin is the smaller, it may be reasonable to consider caesarean section. It is common practice to carry out a caesarean section at 38 weeks in those not suitable for a vaginal delivery, and to induce at 38–40 weeks those who are suitable but have not established labour spontaneously. Some clinicians will electively deliver monochorionic twins preterm.

MANAGEMENT OF TWIN DELIVERY

Labour

Establish IV access and send blood for group and save. An epidural may be very useful in assisting the delivery of a second twin particularly if it is not cephalic. The first stage is managed as for singleton pregnancies. It is useful to confirm the fetal lie, presentation and position of the hearts with ultrasound in early labour. An experienced obstetrician, anaesthetist, two paediatricians and two midwives should be present for delivery, and a Syntocinon infusion should be ready in case uterine activity falls away after delivery of the first twin (there is no literature on the rate of infusion, but starting at 3 mU/min increasing in 30 minutes to 6 mU/min is considered acceptable by many, see p. 91).

After delivery of the first twin it is often helpful to have someone 'stabilize' the second twin by abdominal palpation while a VE is performed to assess the station of the presenting part. If a second bag of membranes is present, it should not be broken until the presenting part has descended into the pelvis. If the second twin lies transverse after the delivery of the first twin, external cephalic or breech version is appropriate. If still transverse (particularly likely if the back is towards the fundus), the choice is between breech extraction (gentle continuous traction on one or both feet through intact membranes) or caesarean section. There is an increased incidence of PPH.

TRIPLETS AND HIGHER MULTIPLES

For those with higher order multiples, reduction to twins at 12–14 weeks may be considered. With quadruplets or greater, there is likely to be overall benefit. For triplets, the situation is less clear. The miscarriage rate is increased (7.6% vs 2.6%) but the number delivering between 24 and 32 weeks is lower (8.2% vs 24.0%). Since severe preterm delivery is associated with risks of neonatal death and severe handicap, reduction to twins may not improve the chance of survival, but may reduce the rate of handicap. Whether these small benefits are justifiable on medical grounds alone, however, is difficult to assess, as a significant proportion of couples suffer long-term guilt. Most clinicians would deliver those with triplets or higher order gestations by caesarean section because of problems with malpresentation and difficulties with intrapartum fetal monitoring.

PLACENTA PRAEVIA AND PAINLESS PV BLEEDING ANTENATALLY

> **Remember:**
> *Never* perform a VE in the presence of PV bleeding without first excluding a praevia. 'No PV until no PP.'
>
> (See also Haemorrhage, p. 106)

There may be minimal or no PV loss in a large abruption and an abruption is usually, but not always, painful. There may be rapid and severe haemorrhage from a placenta praevia.

Placenta praevia

- Minor: — I   encroaches on lower segment
-           II (marginal) reaches internal os.
- Major: — III (partial) covers part of os
-    -   IV (complete).

The incidence increases with maternal age and previous caesarean sections. Two per cent of those with a low-lying placenta before 24 weeks, 5% of those at 24–29 weeks and 23% of those at ≥ 30 weeks will still have a praevia at term. Those with major recurrent bleeds are sometimes managed as inpatients, but most are managed on an outpatient basis with admission for bleeds and elective delivery at 38 weeks' gestation.

Consider delivery of grade I vaginally (engagement of the presenting part is probably more important than the actual distance of placenta from os on USS). Placenta praevia sections should be supervised/performed by a senior obstetrician, particularly if the placenta is anterior, and a large blood loss should be anticipated.

If the placenta invades the myometrium it is termed *placenta accreta*. If it reaches the serosa, it is termed *placenta increta*, and if through the serosa, it is termed *percreta*. The incidence of placenta accreta is higher after previous caesarean sections (see PPH, p. 107).

Painless PV spotting

This is common. Check the patient's history (pain, postcoital, date of last smear) and blood group. Confirm that the uterus is soft (contractions with labour, hard between contractions with abruption) and check for engagement (if engaged, it is not placenta praevia). Arrange an USS to check the placental site (even large abruptions may not be seen on USS) and, providing there is no praevia, use a speculum to look for cervical effacement, dilatation, an ectropion and (only very rarely) carcinoma. If all is normal it is common practice to admit the patient until the bleeding settles. Many clinicians will not admit the patient if the bleeding is slight and is seen to be coming from an ectropion.

POLYHYDRAMNIOS

This may be defined as more than 2–3 litres of amniotic fluid, but for practical clinical purposes may be considered as:

- a single pool > 8 cm
- an amniotic fluid index > 90th centile (Fig. 2.5).

It occurs in 0.5–2% of all pregnancies and is associated with maternal diabetes (≈ 20%) and congenital fetal anomaly (≈ 5%), particularly:

- Obstruction: oesophageal atresia (commonly in tracheo–oesophageal fistula), duodenal atresia (see p. 20), small intestine or colonic obstruction (atresia, Hirschsprung's disease, see p. 33).

- High urine output: macrosomia, recipient of twin–twin transfusion (see p. 63), or placental or fetal tumour.
- Neuromuscular poor swallowing (rare): anencephaly, myotonic dystrophy (see p. 34), maternal myaesthenia, fetal akinesia sequence or spinal muscular atrophy.
- Mechanical (very rare): facial tumour, macroglossia or micrognathia.

Even in the absence of an identifiable cause (> 60%), polyhydramnios is associated with an increased rate of caesarean section, antepartum fetal death (0.6% vs 0.2%), postpartum death (2.8% vs 0.4%), abruption (0.9% vs 0.3%), malpresentation (6.8% vs 2.9%), cord prolapse (2.2% vs 0.3%) and carrying a large-for-gestational age infant (24% vs 8%).

Investigations

- USS (fetal anomaly scan, growth and skeletal survey), GTT, Rhesus status and fetal well-being assessment.

Management

- Conservative management is usual, with amnioreduction only if symptoms very severe.
- Increased antenatal fetal surveillance.
- Awareness of the risks of intrapartum complications.
- Paediatric involvement at delivery.

PRELABOUR RUPTURE OF MEMBRANES (PROM)

Occurs in 6–12% of live births.

TERM

 A digital vaginal examination is not indicated if the mother is not in labour.

- In 70% of cases, rupture of membranes is established in labour by 24 hours and in 90% by 48 hours. Providing, therefore, that the mother is apyrexial, the baby is in cephalic presentation, the liquor is clear and the CTG is normal a case may be made for adopting a conservative policy for 48 hours. There is also evidence, however, that induction of labour on admission may reduce the incidence of neonatal infection with no increase in caesarean section (N Engl J Med 1996:1005). Delivery must be undertaken at once (ideally by caesarean section unless labour is well established) if there is a clinical suspicion of chorioamnionitis with pyrexia or meconium (pain and discharge are late features).

- Accurate diagnosis is vital. Speculum examination is not essential if the diagnosis is obvious, but may be used to take an HVS and to establish the diagnosis by presence of liquor with vernix, meconium or ferning.

PRETERM (< 37 WEEKS)

> ⚠ A digital vaginal examination is not indicated if the mother is not in labour.

- Occurs in 2–3% of all pregnancies but in 40–60% of all preterm deliveries. It is associated with polyhydramnios, twins and infection (especially group B streptococcus, gonococcus, mycoplasma and, rarely, listeria). Up to a third may occur secondary to infection.
- Scan to confirm presentation. The biophysical profile is difficult to interpret without the parameter of liquor volume. Absence of fetal breathing movements *may* indicate infection, but prolonged scanning (> 30 min) may be required.
- Check the temperature, an MSU and the WCC (rises after maternal steroids) ± C-reactive protein (a better predictor of chorioamnionitis, but still with low sensitivity).
- It may be considered appropriate to carry out a sterile speculum examination to take an HVS and to establish the diagnosis (see above), but an HVS is not a predictor of subsequent infection and such procedures may themselves introduce infection.

Management of preterm prelabour rupture of membranes (PPROM).

- Give dexamethasone or betamethasone 24 mg IM over 48 hours if < 34 weeks. There is currently no consensus regarding repeating courses of corticosteroids if the patient remains undelivered > 7 days after the original course.

- Routine antibiotic use appears to delay delivery and reduce major markers of neonatal morbidity. The choice of antibiotic is unclear, but erythromycin 250 mg QID PO is preferable to co-amoxiclav, as this is associated with a slight increase in neonatal necrotizing enterocolitis (Lancet 2001;979:357).

- Most mothers will establish in labour (e.g. ≈ 75% at 28 weeks establish within 7 days). Do not give tocolytics unless contracting and you are certain that there is no chorioamnionitis. There is no evidence that tocolysis is beneficial in the presence of PPROM, and the use of tocolytics can only be justified in highly selected cases.

- Regular fetal monitoring is essential.

- If the mother does not establish in labour, the problem is one of balancing the risks of chorioamnionitis (which accounts for 20% of neonatal deaths) against the risks of delivery. Infection supervenes after membranes have ruptured in 0.5% and 25% of cases, depending on the criteria employed for diagnosis. The incidence increases with the number of VEs performed.

- It is considered acceptable practice to manage these patients on an outpatient basis following an initial inpatient stay; the patient may take her own temperature at home on a QID basis. It is also common practice to deliver if > 36 weeks.

- If infection develops, take blood cultures and give antibiotics (e.g. ampicillin 500 mg IV QID and gentamicin – see dosage p. 129). Deliver ASAP, ideally by caesarean section, unless labour is well established.

- The outcome becomes more guarded the earlier membrane rupture occurs on account of pulmonary hypoplasia and severe skeletal deformities. Pulmonary hypoplasia occurs in 50% with SRM before 20 weeks and 3% after 24 weeks. Lung size, amniotic fluid volume and fetal breathing movements on antenatal ultrasound are not reliable predictors of pulmonary hypoplasia.

PROLONGED PREGNANCY (> 42 WEEKS)

This occurs in 10% of pregnancies and is associated with an increased perinatal mortality (perinatal mortality is 5 : 1000 between 37 and 42 weeks and 9.7 : 1000 after 42 weeks) due to IUD, intrapartum hypoxia and meconium aspiration syndrome. Dating the pregnancy by ultrasound before 18 weeks is more reliable than LMP in reducing the incidence of prolonged pregnancy.

Sweeping the membranes at term is associated with reduced duration of pregnancy and reduced frequency of pregnancy continuing beyond 41 weeks (RR 0.62) and 42 weeks (RR 0.28). This benefit needs to be balanced against women's discomfort (*www.cochrane.co.uk* 2004). The risk of infection is considered to be minimal.

Induction of labour at > 41 weeks reduces the incidence of fetal distress and meconium staining over those managed conservatively with monitoring (N Engl J Med 1996:1005). There is also a reduction in the caesarean section rate and no increase in the incidence of uterine hypertonus. No effect on perinatal mortality has been demonstrated. It has been estimated, however, that 500 inductions may be required to prevent one perinatal death. The ideal timing of induction after 41 weeks is unknown. Dissatisfaction of labour is strongly associated with operative delivery, and is not associated with induction of labour.

The use of ultrasound and CTG in the monitoring of postdates pregnancy confers no demonstrable benefit.

SMALL FETUS (SGA AND IUGR)

> **Small for gestational age (SGA) refers to those fetuses that weigh < 10th centile for gestational age. They may simply be inherently small, but healthy and growing along their centile. Intrauterine growth restriction (IUGR) refers to any fetus failing to achieve its growth potential. Not all small-for-dates (SFD) fetuses are growth restricted, and not all growth-restricted fetuses are SFD.**

The small fetus carries an increased risk of intrauterine death, intrapartum asphyxia, neonatal hypoglycaemia and possible long-term neurological impairment. The perinatal mortality is also higher:

- > 10th centile overall, 12 : 1000
- 5th–10th centile, 22 : 1000
- < 5th centile, 190 : 1000 (80% occur in utero, with 50% of these occurring after 36 weeks).

In theory, a SGA fetus that has a normal growth velocity is likely to be simply inherently small, whereas a baby with IUGR (i.e. reduced growth velocity) should be investigated further. In reality, the two are often initially managed in the same way, as the difference only becomes apparent with time. Risk factors for IUGR include smoking, previous SGA babies and 'unexplained' increased αFP.

Causes of IUGR

- Uteroplacental insufficiency: pre-eclampsia, abruption or unexplained.
- Fetal factors: congenital abnormality (17% in those < 5th centile), congenital infection or in association with multiple pregnancy.
- Maternal factors: smoking, nutrition, alcohol, drugs, Rhesus iso-immunization or medical problems (severe anaemia, or cardiovascular, renal or GI pathology).

Diagnosis

This usually follows antenatal screening. Clinical examination (+/– symphyseal fundal height measurement) has a 30–50% sensitivity of identifying IUGR in a low risk population. While ultrasound measurements perform a little better, they may lead to greater intervention for no demonstrable neonatal benefit (Cochrane 2004).

Management

- History for the above maternal causes.
- BP and urine dipsticks to exclude pre-eclampsia.
- USS for fetal anomaly.

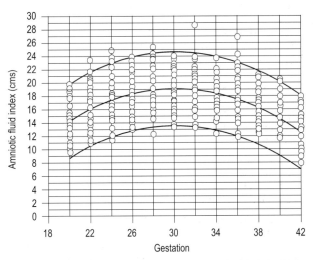

Fig. 2.5 Gestation reference range (mean +/– two standard deviations) for amniotic fluid index. (Reproduced from BJOG 817, 1993, with the permission of the Royal College of Obstetricians and Gynaecologists.)

- Check Doppler studies of the umbilical artery, as well as liquor volume (+/– CTG depending on findings) (see Liquor volume, Fig. 2.5).
- It is usually impossible to minimize causal factors (except smoking).
- Steroids should be given if delivery before 34 weeks is anticipated (see p. 94).

The frequency of monitoring in the non-compromised fetus depends on many factors, but it may be possible to monitor on an outpatient basis every 1–14 days depending on ongoing results (Fig. 2.2). Inpatient monitoring or delivery should be considered if the fetus is compromised. Decisions about the timing and mode of delivery are often difficult and depend on all of the above factors (see also Fetal monitoring, p. 47).

CHAPTER 3

MIDWIFERY SKILLS

PHILOSOPHY OF CARE

The majority of women will progress through pregnancy and labour without the need for intervention. Pregnancy is a normal physiological process and it is hoped that most women will give birth normally. For a physiological process, however, pregnancy is surprisingly hazardous. Worldwide, over half a million women die every year from pregnancy-related causes and many could be saved with the most basic of healthcare provision. Even with the best medical care, however, lives are still lost and there is the temptation in affluent countries to over-medicalize normal pregnancy, perhaps interfering when there are no real problems. Such interference serves to increase the risk of harm. Midwifery therefore faces two challenges: how to provide more effective care in countries with limited resources and how to make our interventions more appropriate in the affluent world. While Chapter 5 considers issues related to less affluent countries, this chapter focuses on midwifery challenges in a western setting.

There is both an art and a science to being a midwife: a sound understanding of the psychology of labour is just as important to a good outcome as a thorough understanding of physiology. Midwifery care should be professional, individualized, and respectful of the mother and her family; it should allow women to be looked after safely and, if possible, to have the opportunity to give birth normally.

Such philosophies, however, are often idealistic. Realistically, women-centred care can be difficult and costly to truly achieve. Nonetheless, midwives almost always make the key difference to a labour through encouragement, and by giving women self-belief in their ability to deliver normally. Normal childbirth is an empowering experience for many women, which in turn expresses itself in their ability to adapt to parenthood and in the care they give their baby.

ANTENATAL CARE

While antenatal care has an important role in screening for obstetric medical problems, it is also an important opportunity to spend time with a couple to build relationships and trust. This familiarity can, in itself, be helpful in recognizing when something is going wrong. Midwives are ideally placed to be the primary care-giver, carrying out ongoing monitoring and assessment throughout the time of pregnancy and childbirth, and referring when problems are identified.

In the course of her pregnancy a women usually sees her midwife regularly from the initial booking visit, with appointments progressing from monthly to fortnightly and then weekly. Checks involve assessing:

- any pre-existing medical conditions
- blood pressure and urinalysis
- fetal growth, presentation, and heartbeat
- mental well-being
- social problems, involving other agencies as appropriate (e.g. social work, physiotherapy)
- child protection issues and drug misuse problems, involving liaison teams if required.

Communication plays a large part in midwifery, requiring skills in counselling and in education where necessary. Many women have a good understanding of the process of pregnancy from previous experience, accounts from friends, television and books. Others, however, need to be given specific information and time should be made for this during visits. Ideally both the woman and her partner should be prepared for the transition from pregnancy to parenthood. Expectations are often high and not always realistic, and the midwife can try to bring the situation back into perspective. She may also provide evidence-based information to help a couple with more difficult choices.

While midwives are ideally placed to lead in normal pregnancy, obstetricians should be seen as the lead professional where problems occur. The roles of midwife and obstetrician are, however, interdependent, with both professionals relying closely on each other.

LABOUR

HOME DELIVERY

Giving birth in relaxed familiar surroundings, where there is privacy, comfort and freedom, and where women feel in control of their labour, is associated with less medical intervention than delivery in a hospital environment. A meta-analysis of observational studies on the safety of home birth (*www.cochrane.co.uk* 2004) showed that fewer medical interventions occurred in home birth groups: less augmentation, fewer episiotomies, less operative vaginal birth and fewer caesarean sections. Furthermore there was a lower frequency of low Apgar scores and severe lacerations. The only RCT on this subject is too small to draw specific conclusions.

Safety is the key question. There is extensive evidence that hospital delivery is safer than home delivery in high-risk pregnancies but the situation is much less clear for those at low risk. It is quite possible that home delivery might carry fewer risks for those that fulfil specific criteria including: a planned home delivery, a well-trained attendant, no medical or obstetric problems, adequate screening, and appropriate facilities to transfer to a nearby hospital. The Netherlands, for example, has a home delivery rate of 35% (the highest percentage of any industrialized nation) and maintains one of the lowest perinatal mortality rates worldwide. There is a high level of maternal satisfaction and the environment often avoids the iatrogenic risks through the excessive use of technology (Clin Obstet Gynecol 2001:676).

Despite this encouraging evidence, there is always the small possibility of an unexpected peripartum emergency. Ideally the final decision should rest with an agreed plan between the parents and their carers. For many mothers and midwives, home birth can be a particularly special experience.

DIAGNOSIS OF LABOUR

It is fundamentally important to appreciate that there is an overwhelming difference between the labour of a primigravida (a mother having her first labour) and that of a parous woman who has had a previous vaginal delivery (Table 3.1). A first labour is one of the most profound emotional experiences any individual will experience. A successful well-managed vaginal delivery first time around usually leads to subsequent deliveries being relatively uneventful. Conversely, a poorly managed first labour can add to subsequent obstetric problems, and have emotional ramifications far beyond any obstetrical complications that may occur.

The initial contact with hospital staff is very important and will dictate immediate care. An error at this stage, medical or social, often leads to later problems in labour. Time spent making a thorough initial assessment is likely to be invaluable:

- Look at the mother: How is she coping? Does she seem distressed?
- Contractions should be assessed on: onset, frequency, strength (by manual palpation), maternal history.
- Vaginal loss: Presence? History of show?
- Rupture of membranes: When? Colour of liquor?

The diagnosis of 'labour' is pivotal to management. The diagnosis is easy in retrospect, but of course a prospective diagnosis is required.

TABLE 3.1 The difference between a normal primigravid and multigravid labour

Primigravida	Multigravida
Unique psychological experience	
Inefficient uterine action common, therefore labour often longer	Uterine action efficient and genital tract stretches more easily, therefore labour usually shorter
The functional capacity of the pelvis is not known. Cephalopelvic disproportion is a possibility	Cephalopelvic disproportion is rare. If it does occur, it is usually secondary to some serious problem
Serious injury to the child relatively more common. The incidence of instrumental delivery is higher	Serious injury to the child is rare. Furthermore, the risk of birth injury is less when the baby is born by propulsion rather than traction
Uterus virtually immune to rupture	There is a small risk of uterine rupture, particularly if there is a pre-existing caesarean section scar

The presence of palpable contractions does not necessarily mean that a woman is in labour, as Braxton Hicks contractions are common antenatally. There has to be contractions together with effacement and dilatation of the cervix.

Effacement has occurred when the entire length of the cervical canal has been taken up into the lower segment of the uterus, a process that begins at the internal os and proceeds downwards to the external os. This is analogous to pulling a polo-necked sweater over one's head. It is of note that 'dilatation' refers only to the dilation of the external os. Again, there is an important difference between primigravid and multigravid labours as dilatation will not begin in a primigravida until effacement has occurred, whereas both may occur simultaneously in a parous woman.

If there are regular contractions and a fully effaced cervix, the woman can be said to be in labour. If, however, there are contractions with only a partially effaced cervix, further objective evidence must be sought in the form of either a 'show' or spontaneous membrane rupture. A 'show', or blood-stained mucous discharge, has occurred in approximately two-thirds of women by the time of presentation and supports the diagnosis *in those with regular contractions*. Spontaneous membrane rupture *in the presence of regular contractions* also confirms the diagnosis.

HELPING THE FIRST STAGE MANAGE ITSELF

'Management of labour' infers that labour is something which is controlled and dictated by the medical or midwifery staff. A straightforward labour, however, should manage itself with midwifery support. Historically, women have been attended and supported by other women during labour but in recent decades in many hospitals, continuous support during labour has become the exception rather than the routine and concerns about the consequent dehumanization of women's birth experiences have led to calls for a return to previous practice. There is good evidence that women who have continuous intrapartum support are less likely to have intrapartum analgesia, an operative birth, or to report dissatisfaction with their childbirth experiences (*www.cochrane.co.uk* 2004).

Team midwifery goes some way to achieving closer care, with midwives carrying a specific caseload and offering both home deliveries and 'domino' (domiciliary in and out, i.e. early labour at home, in to hospital for delivery and home again shortly after). This reduces the number of different midwives a woman may meet during her pregnancy and allows for more choice and trust in the midwife who will eventually deliver her baby. It reflects the common theme that mothers are keen to know the staff who are looking after them in labour, at the time they feel most vulnerable, and they would like to have met them prior to labour. In large units this can often be very difficult to achieve.

The latent phase of labour is said to be when regular contractions occur but the cervix is not yet effaced or dilated. Many women present at this point and such contractions can last for hours or even days. For many women simply seeing a midwife either at home or in hospital is enough support, and it is important to encourage mobility, continue normal diet and fluids and consider non-pharmacological methods of pain relief (water, heat, massage, reflexology, etc). Opiates can be used, but may cause drowsiness and have a 'hangover' effect which can affect a woman's ability to cope with her ensuing labour.

It is just as important to recognize when a woman is in active labour as it is not uncommon for women to labour undetected, and sudden delivery at home, in the car or before reaching the labour ward can be emotionally traumatic.

Preparing a mother for the length of labour is critically important. When working in a shift system there can be a tendency to tide someone over until the end of that shift rather than to follow the pace of labour itself. Caesarean section in the first stage of labour can be difficult to avoid if a mother has prepared herself for delivery by a certain time and, even though progress is good and vaginal delivery probable, she reaches the specified time undelivered. It may therefore be useful to be pessimistic about time in early labour rather than have the midwife on the next shift being faced with a disappointed and distrustful mother.

The decision about when to call the doctor for support is a difficult one and depends on the seriousness of the problem and the experience of the midwife. Calling too early alleviates the midwife of her anxiety and responsibility, and may be medico-legally safer for her. At the same time, however, she risks bringing in someone who may be less experienced than she is, and who is familiar with 'abnormality' rather than 'normality'. This may not necessarily be the most appropriate way to achieve a vaginal delivery. Calling too late, however, may expose the mother and her baby to undue risks. Asking for appropriate help at the right time is the hallmark of experience.

ANALGESIA

Pain relief is discussed in detail on page 96. Metanalysis of randomized trials suggests that use of epidural anaesthesia does not increase the rate of caesarean section, but does increase the risk of instrumental delivery (BMJ 2004:1410). Epidural use is not associated with long-term backache in comparison to those who do not have one (BMJ 2002:357).

COMPLEMENTARY THERAPY IN LABOUR

Complementary medicine is the treatment and prevention of disease by techniques regarded by Western medicine as scientifically unproven or unorthodox. While sceptics argue that any apparent benefits are simply the effect of placebo, others believe that many therapies have important roles, and some encouraging research is beginning to emerge. A few of these complementary techniques are used in labour and are outlined below.

Homeopathy dates from the early 19th century and is a system of medicine in which the fundamental principle is the law of similars, in that 'like' is cured by 'like'. When a drug was found to produce the same symptoms as did a certain disease, it was then used in much smaller doses to treat that disease. It had been observed, for example, that quinine given to a healthy person caused similar symptoms to those of malaria and quinine therefore became a treatment for malaria. The principle of homeopathy is that the smaller the dose, the greater the effect, and most potencies are administered in such minute doses as to contain less than a small number of molecules, if any at all.

Acupuncture is a technique of traditional Chinese medicine dating back 5000 years in which a number of very fine metal needles are inserted into the skin at specifically designated points. These points are not distributed at random but follow a prescribed pattern, and the lines that link these points to each organ system are referred to as meridians. Research has suggested that acupuncture may work by stimulating or repressing the autonomic nervous system, and may affect endorphin release. It has been used extensively antenatally with some success, as well as for induction of labour and for pain relief in labour itself.

Herbal medicine, the use of natural plant substances to treat disease, has existed since prehistoric times and is the primary form of medicine for around 80% of the world's population. Over 80 000 species of plants are regarded as having useful properties. Use in obstetrics, including labour, is widespread but there is little supportive research to suggest benefit or otherwise. Caution is always required in administering any preparation in pregnancy that may carry the potential for adverse fetal affects.

Other techniques include hypnosis, reflexology, massage treatments and various 'new age therapies' such as guided imagery and naturopathy.

CTGS

Cerebral palsy is often the result of antenatal factors rather than intrapartum problems. This, however, should not be an excuse for careless intrapartum care and every effort should still be made to identify and act upon identifiable causes of potential cerebral injury. Despite meta-analysis involving over 1500 pregnancies, however, there are insufficient data to properly evaluate the use of antenatal cardiotocography as a method of avoiding intrapartum injury (*www.cochrane.co.uk* 2004). In particular, the use of cardiotocography has been shown to increase the rate of obstetric intervention. Any interpretation of a CTG has to take account the full clinical situation rather than just the isolated CTG itself. Meconium staining of the liquor, for example, increases the chance that there is underlying fetal compromise but a normal CTG is usually reassuring. Guidelines for the use of CTGs are summarized in Figure 3.1.

It is common practice to administer maternal oxygen if there is a non-reassuring pattern. This has not been shown to be of benefit, and indeed there is a possibility that it may be harmful to the fetus (*www.cochrane.co.uk* 2004).

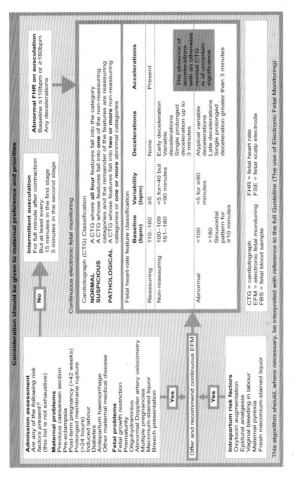

Consideration should be given to maternal preference and priorities

Admission assessment
Are any of the following risk factors present?
(this list is not exhaustive)

Maternal problems
Previous caesarean section
Pre-eclampsia
Post-term pregnancy (>42 weeks)
Prolonged membrane rupture (>24 hours)
Induced labour
Diabetes
Antepartum haemorrhage
Other maternal medical disease

Fetal problems
Fetal growth restriction
Prematurity
Oligohydramnios
Abnormal Doppler artery velocimetry
Multiple pregnancies
Meconium-stained liquor
Breech presentation

No → **Intermittent auscultation**
For full minute after contraction
But at least every:
15 minutes in the first stage
5 minutes in the second stage

Abnormal FHR on auscultation
Baseline ≤110bpm or ≥160bpm
Any decelerations

Yes → Offer and recommend continuous EFM

Intrapartum risk factors
Oxytocin augmentation
Epidural analgesia
Vaginal bleeding in labour
Maternal pyrexia
Fresh meconium-stained liquor

Yes → Continuous electronic fetal monitoring

Cardiotograph (CTG) Classification

NORMAL A CTG where **all four** features fall into the category
SUSPICIOUS A CTG whose features fall into **one** of the non-reassuring catagories and the remainder of the features are reassuring
PATHOLOGICAL A CTG whose features fall into **two or more** non-reassuring catagories or **one or more** abnormal catagories

Fetal heart-rate feature classification

	Baseline (bpm)	Variability (bpm)	Decelerations	Accelerations
Reassuring	110–160	≥5	None	Present
Non-reassuring	100–109 161–180	<5 for 40 but <90 minutes	Early deceleration Variable decelerations Single prolonged deceleration up to 3 minutes	The absence of accelerations with an otherwise normal CTG is of uncertain significance
Abnormal	<100 >180 Sinusoidal pattern for ≥10 minutes	<5 for ≥90 minutes	Atypical variable decelerations Late decelerations Single prolonged deceleration greater than 3 minutes	

CTG = cardiotograph
EFM = electronic fetal monitoring
FBS = fetal blood sample

FHR = fetal heart rate
FSE = fetal scalp electrode

This algorithm should, where necessary, be interpreted with reference to the full Guideline (The use of Electronic Fetal Monitoring)

Fig.3.1 Electronic fetal monitoring. (Adapted from NICE guidelines.)

WATER LABOUR

Enthusiasts for immersion in water during labour, and birth, have advocated its use to increase maternal relaxation, reduce analgesia requirements and promote a more positive birth experience. Many mothers feel that their experience is one of a more gentle delivery. Sceptics, on the other hand, are concerned that there may be a risk to the baby from inhaling the water. Randomized evidence concludes that water *labour* reduces the use of analgesia but there is no significant difference in the vaginal delivery rate, Apgar scores, neonatal admissions or neonatal infections. Mothers using water pools report less pain than those not labouring in water (*www.cochrane.co.uk* 2004). There are only very limited data on water *birth*, but observational work is reassuring (BMJ 1999:483).

SECOND STAGE

There has long been controversy about whether being upright in labour (sitting, birthing stools, chairs, squatting) has advantage over lying down. Meta-analysis suggests very little difference between either group, with perhaps a very tentative benefit from the upright position (*www.cochrane.co.uk* 2004).

Opinions differ about whether women should be asked to push when they are found to be fully dilated, or whether they should wait 1–2 hours to allow the head to descend (passive second stage) before then starting to push (active second stage). Objective evidence is equivocal. There is work to suggest that a passive second stage in those with an epidural is associated with a shorter time of pushing, fewer CTG decelerations and less fatigue than those with no passive time, but there is no difference in fetal outcome, instrumental delivery rates or short-term perineal injury (Obstet Gynecol 2002:29).

There is also no clear consensus as to the appropriate length of the second stage. While very long second stages are associated with vesico–vaginal fistulae and other longer-term perineal problems, it is common for the second stage to last quite a few hours with no apparent problems.

There is evidence that early skin to skin contact (contact with the mother's bare chest at birth or at least within the first 24 hours) may represent a 'sensitive period' for priming mothers and infants to develop a synchronous, reciprocal, interaction pattern. It is likely that this facilitates subsequent successful breast-feeding and that these babies cry less (*www.cochrane.co.uk* 2004).

EPISIOTOMY

It was previously felt that the use of episiotomy reduced the incidence of anal sphincter tears. There is, however, little good evidence to support this and there is certainly no evidence to support routine episiotomy in all deliveries as a preventative measure against third or fourth degree tears. Midline episiotomy in particular does not protect the perineum or sphincters during childbirth and may impair anal continence. If an episiotomy is to be performed at all, a right (or less commonly left) posterolateral episiotomy is preferred.

The rate of episiotomy has wide geographic variations from 8% in the Netherlands, to 20% in the UK, 50% in the USA and 99% in some eastern European countries. It is also high in many developing countries. Defining a 'good' episiotomy rate is therefore difficult. Restricting the use of episiotomy to specific fetal and maternal indications leads to lower rates of posterior perineal trauma, less need for suturing and fewer long-term complications (*www.cochrane.co.uk* 2004). A tear may be less painful than an episiotomy and may also heal better.

Possible indications for an episiotomy:

- a rigid perineum which is preventing delivery
- if it is felt that a large tear is imminent
- most instrumental deliveries (forceps or ventouse)
- shoulder dystocia
- breech delivery.

The continuous subcuticular technique of perineal repair may be associated with less pain in the immediate postpartum period than the interrupted suture technique. The long-term effects are less clear.

THIRD STAGE

Expectant management of the third stage of labour involves allowing the placenta to deliver spontaneously or aiding it by gravity or nipple stimulation. Active management involves administration of a prophylactic oxytocic before delivery of the placenta and controlled cord traction of the umbilical cord (often with early cord clamping and cutting). Routine 'active management' is considerably superior to 'expectant management' in terms of blood loss, postpartum haemorrhage and other serious complications of the third stage of labour. Active management is, however, associated with an increased risk of unpleasant side-effects (e.g. nausea and vomiting), and hypertension, where ergometrine is used. Active management should be the routine management of choice for women expecting to deliver a baby by vaginal delivery in a maternity hospital.

POSTNATAL CARE

> **This is a time of great change. Women are adjusting to their new role, getting to know their baby and learning to be a parent. During the early neonatal period, midwives screen for potential complications like anaemia, vaginal bleeding (heavy suggests retained tissue), perineal breakdown, bladder or bowel dysfunction, feeding problems and pyrexia (suggests infection, e.g. UTI or occasionally venous thromboembolic problems).**

Supportive help with breast-feeding is also important; this has been shown to improve breast-feeding success rates (*www.cochrane.co.uk* 2004). Breast engorgement can occur on the second or third day as the milk supply comes in and can be very uncomfortable, causing problems with fixing the baby to the nipple. Women can be shown how to hand express and how to use warm/cold flannels for comfort until regular feeding is established. Supplementation should ideally be avoided. Artificial feeding is still the method of choice for some women and advice can be given on frequency, volumes and preparation of feeds.

Postnatal emotional issues are discussed on page 196, and midwives are aware of the need to look out for these problems. Encouragement is vital, particularly as this is an exceptionally exhausting time. It is also a useful opportunity to consider postnatal depression, although formal routine screening for low risk women is unlikely to be helpful (*www.sign.ac.uk*).

Finally, contraception should be planned and arranged according to individual preferences and suitability.

CHAPTER 4

ACUTE OBSTETRICS AND RELATED MEDICAL PROBLEMS

ACUTE OBSTETRICS

NORMAL LABOUR

> Normal labour begins spontaneously at 37–42 weeks,
> progresses at an acceptable rate (see below) and results in the
> spontaneous vaginal delivery of a live undistressed neonate in
> the occipitoanterior position.

The first stage is from the onset of labour until full dilatation of the
cervix. Onset may be, but does not need to be, preceded by a show
(mucus or small amount of blood-stained discharge), and true labour
is said to have begun when there is both regular uterine activity and
cervical dilatation. There may be an initial and sometimes prolonged
(hours or days) latent phase before true labour begins, but an
acceptable rate of dilatation after 3 cm is 1 cm/h in a primigravida and
1–2 cm/h in a multigravida. SRM may occur prior to the onset of
labour (see p. 67), but more usually some time after contractions have
started. The head usually engages at the pelvic brim in the
occipitotransverse position (see Fig. 4.2a), flexing as it descends into
the pelvic cavity and rotating to occipitoanterior at the level of the
ischial spines. Progress should be charted on a partogram (Fig. 4.1)
together with maternal pulse, blood pressure, temperature, fetal heart
rate, cervical dilatation, descent of the presenting part, frequency of
contractions and presence or absence of meconium. It is reasonable to
carry out a vaginal examination at least every 4 hours to assess
dilatation, descent (relative to ischial spines), position, caput and
moulding (1 if the sutures are aligned, 2 if overlapping, 3 if
irreducible). In low-risk mothers the fetal heart rate may be monitored
either intermittently (approximately every 15 minutes, with a reading
taken before, during and after a contraction) or continuously with a
cardiotocograph (see p. 98).

The second stage is from full dilatation until delivery of the baby
(Fig. 4.2 b–e). There may be an initial passive (non-pushing) phase
before the desire to push is felt, followed by an active (pushing) stage.
The head extends as it descends, distending the vulva until it is
delivered. It then externally rotates to the transverse position again as
the shoulders are rotated within the pelvis to the AP plane and the
anterior shoulder is delivered by downward lateral traction of the
trunk, with subsequent upward lateral traction being used for the
posterior shoulder. The rest of the baby usually follows without

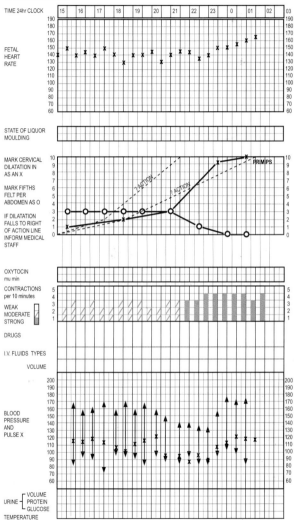

START PARTOGRAM AT CERVICAL DILATION AT FIRST VE PLOTTED ONTO APPROPRIATE POINT ON LINE
TIME PARTOGRAM STARTED

Fig. 4.1 Partogram for primigravid labour. The partogram graph for parous labour is steeper (see text).

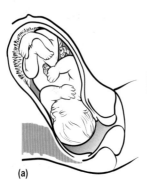

(a)

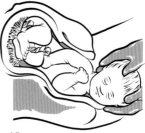

(d)

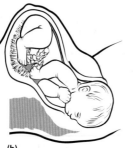

(b)

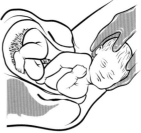

(e)

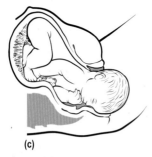

(c)

Fig. 4.2 **(a)** Full dilatation. **(b)** Descent of the head with extension and rotation of the head. **(c)** The shoulders remain behind the symphysis pubis. **(d)** External rotation of the head and delivery of the anterior shoulder. **(e)** Delivery of the posterior shoulder.

difficulty. Normal time for the second stage is 1–3 hours in a primigravida and 1 hour or less in a multigravida.

The third stage is from delivery of the baby until delivery of the placenta. The uterus contracts, shearing the placenta from the uterine wall; this separation is often indicated by a small rush of dark blood and a lengthening of cord. The placenta can then be delivered by gentle cord traction (see Retained placenta), but caution is required to avoid uterine inversion (see p. 123).

The routine use of Syntometrine IM (Syntocinon 5 units and ergotomine 0.5 mg) following delivery of the anterior shoulder reduces the risk of PPH over those managed expectantly in the third stage. It is also probably more effective than Syntocinon alone but it is associated with more nausea and vomiting.

INDUCTION AND AUGMENTATION OF LABOUR

> **Induction of labour refers only to a mother not in labour. Augmentation is the process of accelerating progress after labour has begun.**

Induction

The main risks are of inappropriate use, hyperstimulation and failed induction. Review the gestation, indication and presentation, and assess the cervix using the modified Bishop's Scoring System (Table 4.1). Caution is required with previous caesarean section, previous precipitate labour, or if highly parous. Monitor with CTG at least before induction and as soon as there is uterine activity.

- If the score is < 7, 'ripen' the cervix with prostaglandin E_2 (gel or vaginal tablets).
- If the score is > 7, consider either prostaglandin E_2 or ARM ± Syntocinon (there may be greater patient satisfaction with the former, but the latter may allow more control).

Prostaglandins
The prostaglandins are inserted into the posterior fornix (NICE 2001) as follows:

PGE2 gels
- 2 mg in nulliparous women with an unfavourable cervix (Bishop's score < 4).
- 1 mg for all other women.

TABLE 4.1 Bishop's scoring system for cervical assessment

Score	0	1	2	3
Cervical dilatation (cm)	< 1	1–2	2–4	> 4
Length of cervix (cm)	> 4	2–4	1–2	< 1
Station of presenting part (cm)	Spines –3	Spines –2	Spines –1	At or below spines
Consistency	Firm	Average	Soft	
Position	Posterior	Central	Anterior	

- In either, a second dose of 1–2 mg can be administered 6 hours later providing there is minimal uterine activity.
- The maximum quoted dose is 4 mg for nulliparous women beginning with an unfavourable cervix and 3 mg for all other women.

PGE2 vaginal tablets

- 3 mg, repeated 6–8 hourly providing there is minimal uterine activity.
- The maximum quoted dose is 6 mg for all women.

If at any stage the Bishop's score is > 6, consider an ARM, reassess 2 hours later and start Syntocinon if there is still no change.

Sustained-release preparations are also available. Propess is a polymer-based vaginal insert with retrieval thread containing 10 mg PGE$_2$. It is placed in the posterior fornix for 12 hours (only 5 mg prostaglandin is released over this time), after which it is removed. This technique has the advantage that the insert can be removed if hyperstimulation develops, and trials indicate that it is probably safe. It has not been shown to be superior to gel or tablets.

Artificial rupture of membranes (ARM)

ARM (amniotomy) is used to induce labour in those with a sufficiently favourable cervix and is also used for augmentation (see below). Further, it allows assessment of the colour of the liquor (see Meconium, p. 103). Its routine use in early labour is surrounded by a degree of controversy: it may reduce the duration of labour, but there is a trend towards increasing the caesarean section rate (*www.cochrane.co.uk* 2004).

Early ARM and Syntocinon probably do not confer benefit over conservative management in nulliparous women with mild delays in early spontaneous labour. The fetal head should be well applied to the

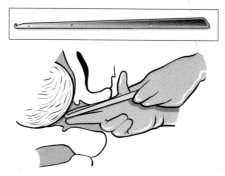

Fig. 4.3 Artificial rupture of the membranes (ARM).

cervix to minimize the risk of cord prolapse. With asepsis, the tips of the index and middle fingers of one hand should be placed through the cervix onto the membranes (Fig. 4.3). An amniotomy hook can then be slid down the groove between these fingers (the hook pointing downwards towards the fingers) until the cervix is reached. The point is then turned upwards to break the membrane sac. Liquor is usually seen, but may be absent in oligohydramnios or with a well-engaged head. Exclude cord prolapse before removing fingers. Check the FH. Absent liquor following ARM should be treated as meconium staining until proven otherwise.

Syntocinon

This may be used for induction following ARM with a favourable cervix, or for augmentation of a slow, non-obstructed labour. It should only be started if the membranes have been ruptured, and continuous CTG monitoring is important. Make up a 1000 ml infusion of 0.9% saline (or Hartmann's solution) with 20 U of Syntocinon (3 ml = 1 mU/min). The dose should be titrated against the contractions, aiming for not more than 6–7 every 15 minutes. Start at 3 ml/h (1 mU/min), increasing every 30 minutes by 3 ml/h until at 24 ml/h. Then increase by 6 ml/h every 30 min to 36 ml/h (12 mU/min). The maximum dose should not exceed 32 mU/min (NICE 2001).

For induction, the use of Syntocinon immediately following ARM reduces the time to delivery, the rates of PPH and the need for operative delivery. As labour will begin within 24 hours in 88% of cases, however, it is unclear whether these advantages outweigh the maternal inconvenience of an IV infusion, restricted mobility and continuous fetal monitoring. An individual approach is advised.

Augmentation

The cause of failure to progress must be considered carefully.

Obstruction may be caused by the baby being too big or the pelvis too small (true cephalopelvic disproportion) or by malposition (relative cephalopelvic disproportion). There may be a clinical suspicion from abdominal palpation, and there is likely to be caput or moulding at VE.

Inadequate dilatation may also be due to inadequate contractions. 'Adequacy' of contractions is very difficult to assess, and some degree of judgement rests with experience and the absence of any evidence of obstruction. If there is felt to be true poor uterine activity it is reasonable to start Syntocinon cautiously, as above. The use of Syntocinon in obstructed labour may lead to uterine rupture.

PRETERM LABOUR

> **This is defined as labour occurring at 24–37 weeks. It occurs in 6–10% of pregnancies, and in about 30% of cases is due to direct medical intervention. Although it may be associated with multiple pregnancy, APH, IUGR, cervical incompetence, amnionitis, congenital uterine anomaly, polyhydramnios or systemic infection, particularly pyelonephritis, many cases are 'idiopathic'.**

There have been a number of techniques proposed to screen for preterm labour. A cervical length of < 15 mm at 23 weeks (measured by TV USS) occurs in 2% of the population but accounts for 90% and 60% of those who will deliver at ≤ 28 and ≤ 32 weeks respectively. The risk of preterm labour with a cervical length of 15 mm is 4%, rising to 78% at a length of < 5 mm (Fig. 4.4). The value of this knowledge is unclear as it remains unknown, for example, whether a cervical suture is indicated, is of no help, or is even contraindicated in such circumstances.

The presence of fetal fibronectin measured on cervical testing is also used in some centres. In those suspected to be in preterm labour, a positive test has a PPV of over 70% depending on gestation, and < 3% of mothers with a negative test will deliver in the subsequent 3 weeks (BJOG 2003;Suppl 20) Its main use may be in the reassurance of a negative test. Benefit from screening for any of the above has not been shown.

Screening for infection has also been considered, but again no benefits have been demonstrated. Bacterial vaginosis, which is present

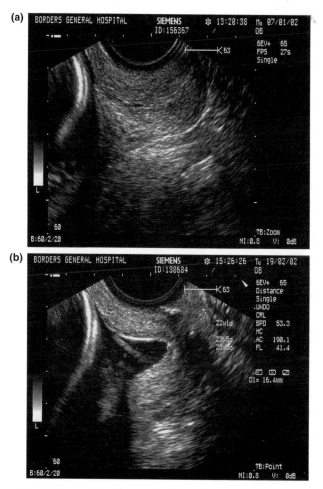

Fig. 4.4 Pre-term labour is unusual in those with a long closed cervix **(a)** as measured by transvaginal scan early in the second trimester. If the cervix is shortened and funnelled **(b)**, there is a much greater chance of preterm labour.

in 10–20% of pregnant women, has been associated with a two-fold relative risk of preterm delivery. There is no benefit from screening low-risk mothers, but treating such an infection in those with a history of preterm labour might be appropriate (*www.cochrane.co.uk* 2004).

Assessment and management

- Is preterm labour likely? Are there palpable contractions (you may need to sit and palpate the uterus)? Is the cervix closed (avoid VE if SRM)?
- Assess fetal and maternal state. Is there evidence of maternal haemorrhage or pyrexia? Is the fetus in cephalic presentation? Is an FH present? CTG if > approx. 28 weeks.
- Alert paediatricians and arrange in utero transfer if necessary.
- Give steroids. These should be given if delivery before 34 weeks is likely. Use betamethasone or dexamethasone 24 mg IM in divided doses over 24 hours. This significantly reduces the incidence of respiratory distress syndrome (by ≈ 50%), necrotizing enterocolitis and periventricular haemorrhage. There is debate about steroid use in those 34–37 weeks pregnant, but note that 94 women in this group will need to be treated to prevent 1 case of RDS (compared with 5 : 1 at 31 weeks). The possibility of unrecognized long-term effects has not been completely excluded. There is no identifiable increase in the incidence of maternal or fetal infection, but steroids are contraindicated with active maternal septicaemia/TB. It is unknown whether it is appropriate to prescribe repeat doses (e.g. 12 mg every 10 days) if delivery risk is still present. Great caution is required when prescribing steroids for those with IDDM as they may lead to secondary hyperglycaemia and possible DKA (IV control with insulin and dextrose may be appropriate).
- There is evidence that antibiotics should not be routinely prescribed for women in spontaneous preterm labour without evidence of clinical infection. (Lancet 2001;989:357).

Consider tocolytics. It may be reasonable not to use a tocolytic as there is no clear evidence that outcome is improved. Tocolysis should be considered if the few days gained could be put to good use such as completing a course of corticosteroids or in utero transfer (RCOG 2002).

- **Atosiban** (Tractocile) is an oxytocin antagonist. It has been shown to reduce the proportion of deliveries within the first 48 hours although, in common with all tocolytics, it has not been shown to be of benefit in terms of improved fetal morbidity or mortality. It is given as an initial bolus of 6.75 mg IV over 1 minute, followed by an IVI at 18 mg/hour for 3 hours, and then at 6 mg/hour for up to 45 hours. Side-effects are uncommon.

- **Ritodrine** (Yutopar) IV is probably similar to Atosiban in efficacy, but has significantly more side effects and therefore should only be considered if Atosiban is unavailable. There have been a number of maternal deaths associated with ritodrine (particularly when also used with steroids), and it must be used under close direct supervision. It is contraindicated with maternal cardiac disease and hyperthyroidism.

The side-effects include maternal and fetal tachycardia (keep maternal P < 140 bpm) and pulmonary oedema. Rarely, severe maternal bradycardia, hypotension and arrhythmias may occur (especially SVT, AF and premature ventricular contractions) as well as visual disturbances, skin flushing, nausea, vomiting, hyperkalaemia and hyperglycaemia (therefore caution with IDDM and potassium sparing diuretics). Monitor the P and BP frequently (e.g. every 15 min), glucose and U&E (e.g. 4 hourly). Keep an accurate fluid balance and auscultate the bases (e.g. 4 hourly).

Ritodrine is supplied in ampoules (50 mg in 5 ml). For an infusion, add three ampoules (i.e. 15 ml, 150 mg drug) to 35 ml of 5% dextrose in a 50 ml syringe (1 ml/h = 50 µg/min). Start infusing at 1 ml/h, increasing by 1 ml/h every 15 min to a maximum of 7 ml/h (350 µg/min). When contractions stop (or if the maternal pulse is > 140 bpm) reduce by 1 ml/h every 30 min. If pulmonary oedema develops, stop the infusion, give O_2, sit the patient up, give furosemide (frusemide) 50 mg IV and morphine 10 mg IV. If there is an arrhythmia, stop the infusion, and check the potassium level.

- **Nifedipine** (30 mg PO BD followed by 20 mg PO 8 hourly) is a potentially useful alternative. It has fewer side effects than ritodrine and may be more effective in delaying delivery.
- **Indometacin** (100 mg suppository OD PR). Trials have shown that this drug may be effective but there are concerns about closure of the fetal ductus arteriosis, impaired fetal renal function, bronchopulmonary dysplasia and persistent pulmonary hypertension in the neonatal period. It may lead to maternal GI irritation, peptic ulceration, thrombocytopenia, allergic reactions, headaches and dizziness.

Cervical cerclage
Elective transvaginal cervical cerclage may be of benefit in those with a history of cervical incompetence, particularly those with a history of more than two deliveries before 37 weeks (BJOG 1993:516). Pooled data, however, remain inconclusive, irrespective of cervical length on

transvaginal scan (*www.cochrane.co.uk* 2004). Transabdominal cervicoisthmic cerclage is a specialist procedure reserved for failed transcervical cerclage.

'Rescue' cerclage refers to the emergency use of a suture in early preterm labour thought to be due to cervical incompetence, and may be used following the reduction of prolapsed membranes.

PRECIPITATE LABOUR

> **This occurs especially with induction of labour, augmentation and grand multiparity.**

Management

- Stop Syntocinon if an infusion is running.
- Give terbutaline 0.25 mg S/C stat.
- Assess the fetal condition:
  - if there is acute 'distress', perform a VE and consider if vaginal delivery is possible
  - if a caesarean section is considered, re-examine the patient in theatre immediately prior to starting (vaginal delivery may be possible).

ANALGESIA FOR LABOUR

> **Antenatal relaxation training may engender calm, thus conserving energy. False expectations may induce distrust.**

Psychological methods

Randomized trials confirm that good support by a trained care-giver can reduce analgesia requirements. Although unsupported by trials, warm-water massage, transcutaneous electrical nerve stimulation (TENS), acupuncture, aromatherapy and reflexology are favoured by some (see page 79).

Systemic opioid analgesia

Pethidine 50–150 mg IM is favoured by many and, although it does not reduce the pain score in labour, many women feel that they mind the pain less. Some women feel disorientated and experience loss of control. Babies may require naloxone immediately postnatally.

Diamorphine 5–10 mg IM is popular in some centres. It is good practice to prescribe an antiemetic at the same time.

Inhalational analgesia

Entonox is a 50% nitrous oxide 50% oxygen mixture. It is probably more effective overall than pethidine, although has little effect on pain score and may make women light-headed and nauseated.

Regional analgesia

This is particularly valuable for prolonged or complicated labour (including twins) and for caesarean sections or instrumental delivery. Anaesthetic experience is essential:

- *Epidural*. A cannula is placed in the extradural space for repeated or continuous infusion of local anaesthetic, blocking the spinal nerves from the uterus and birth canal (T10–L1). It is the only form of labour analgesia to produce consistent reduction in the pain score, but it has potential problems:
  — Maternal problems: occasional failure to establish a block (total or partial); total spinal block; inadvertent spinal block; epidural haematomas.
  — Fetal problems: hypotension, leading to fetal compromise.
- *Spinal analgesia* (a single injection of local anaesthetic into the subarachnoid space) provides a dense block for 2–4 hours which is particularly useful for caesarean section or some instrumental deliveries.

Regional analgesia is contraindicated with a bleeding diathesis (including full anticoagulation), infection or hypovolaemia. It is likely to reduce the second stage desire to push, and may increase the need for instrumental delivery.

> ⚠ If hypotension occurs secondary to distal vasodilation, ensure that the patient is on her side (or at least has 45° of lateral tilt). Take a 30 mg ampoule of ephedrine (1 ml) and dilute to 10 ml with normal saline (i.e. 3 mg/ml). Give 1 ml IV stat. and titrate the dose thereafter according to the response. There may be rebound hypertension.

FETAL MONITORING

> Always consider the background of previous fetal monitoring,
> gestation, growth, meconium and rate of progress in labour.
> If there is acute fetal distress, stop any Syntocinon, turn the
> mother onto her side, give O_2 and check the BP.

Intermittent monitoring

Assessment of the fetal heart rate can be used to provide some
information about fetal well-being. In 'low-risk' labours (see below),
providing an admission CTG is normal, it is probably safe to
auscultate the fetal heart every 15 minutes before and after a
contraction in the first stage and every 5 minutes in the second stage.
A baseline tachycardia or bradycardia, or late decelerations (i.e.
occurring after a contraction) are indications for further evaluation,
often continuous CTG monitoring ± FBS ± intervention. The routine
use of continuous CTG monitoring in low-risk labours may increase
the rate of intervention for no demonstrable fetal benefit.

Continuous heart rate monitoring (CTG) (Fig. 4.5)

> A cardiotocograph measures fetal heart rate together with the
> timing of contractions. All those with risk factors (including
> IUGR, meconium, Syntocinon, epidurals and previous
> caesarean sections) should probably have continuous CTG
> monitoring. Check that you are looking at the correct
> patient's trace and that the paper speed is correct (1 cm/min).
> Intrapartum CTGs are used to screen those who may need
> further assessment (e.g. FBS ± intervention).

CTG with abdominal (Doppler) probe (Tables 4.2, 4.3)

Use DARTH VADER for thorough CTG evaluation:

D	details (name, time, etc.)	**V**	variability
A	assess quality	**A**	accelerations
R	recorded fetal movements	**D**	decelerations
T	tocograph	**E**	evaluation
H	heart rate	**R**	response

Heartrate baseline 110–160 bpm tachycardia is associated with
prematurity, fetal acidosis, maternal pyrexia, and the use of

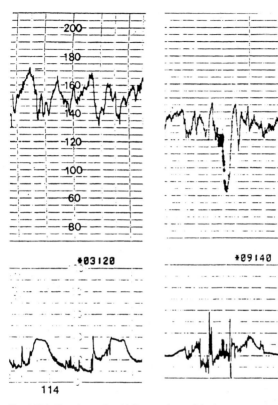

Fig. 4.5(a) There is good variability, but the baseline is difficult to determine.

Fig. 4.5(b) There is an early deceleration on the background of a 140 bpm baseline, with good variability and shouldering.

β-sympathomimetics. Baseline bradycardia is rarely associated with fetal acidosis (unless severe, e.g. abruption or uterine rupture) and is more commonly found with maturity, hypotension, sedation and, rarely, congenital heart block. Cardiac dysrhythmias are rare but can cause extremes of heart rate, either fast or slow, with tachycardia being the more sinister.

Variability This gives the best indication of well-being, normal variability being 5–15 bpm. The commonest reason for loss of baseline variability is the 'sleep' or 'quiet' phase of the fetal

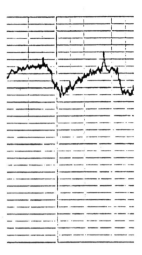
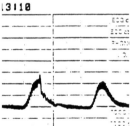
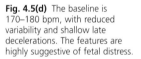
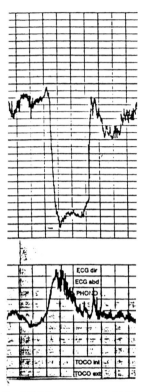
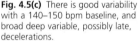

Fig. 4.5(c) There is good variability with a 140–150 bpm baseline, and broad deep variable, possibly late, decelerations.

Fig. 4.5(d) The baseline is 170–180 bpm, with reduced variability and shallow late decelerations. The features are highly suggestive of fetal distress.

behavioural cycle, which may last up to 40 minutes. Loss of variability is also associated with prematurity, acidosis and drugs (e.g. opiates or benzodiazepines). Reduced variability in the presence of late decelerations markedly increases the likelihood of fetal acidosis.

Accelerations These are > 15 bpm and are reassuring.

Decelerations These are of at least 15 bpm and last for more than 15 seconds. Early decelerations occur with contractions. If they occur more than 15 seconds after the contraction they are termed 'late'. 'Variable' contractions vary in both timing and shape.

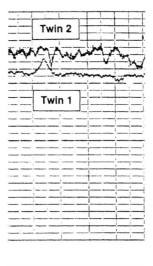

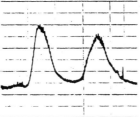

Fig. 4.5(e) Some CTG monitors will add 20 bpm to the baseline of one twin to differentiate it from the other trace. There is reduced variability in twin 1, and the apparent acceleration does not fulfil the criteria for a true acceleration of 15 bpm.

- *Early decelerations* reflect increased vagal tone (intracranial pressure rises during a contraction) and are physiological.
- *Variable decelerations* may represent cord compression (e.g. in oligohydramnios) or acidosis. A small acceleration at the beginning and end of a deceleration (shouldering) suggest that the fetus is coping well with cord compression.
- *Late decelerations* suggest acidosis. Shallow late decelerations may be particularly ominous.

A true sinusoidal trace is rare. There is a smooth undulating sine-wave-like baseline with no variability. It may represent anaemia

TABLE 4.2 Categorization of fetal heart rate (FHR) features (NICE 2001)

Feature	Baseline (bpm)	Variability (bpm)	Decelerations	Accelerations
Reassuring	110–160	= > 5	None	Present
Non-reassuring	100–109 161–180	< 5 for ≥ 40 to < 90 minutes	Early deceleration Variable deceleration Single prolonged deceleration up to 3 minutes	The absence of accelerations with an otherwise normal CTG are of uncertain significance
Abnormal	< 100 > 180 Sinusoidal pattern > = 10 minutes	<5 for >= 90 minutes	Atypical variable decelerations Late decelerations Single prolonged deceleration > 3 minutes	

TABLE 4.3 Categorization of fetal heart rate traces	
Category	Definition
Normal	A CTG where all four features fall into the reassuring category
Suspicious	A CTG whose features fall into one of the non-reassuring categories and the remainder of the features are reassuring
Pathological	A CTG whose features fall into two or more non-reassuring categories or one or more abnormal categories

(especially with an amplitude > 20 bpm at 1–2 oscillations/min) but can be a feature of fetal physiological behaviour. It should be considered to be serious until proven otherwise.

In cases where the CTG falls into the pathological category, fetal blood sampling should be undertaken where appropriate/feasible. In situations where fetal blood sampling is not possible or appropriate, delivery should be expedited.

CTG with scalp clip (Fig. 4.6)

These are used to improve the quality of CTG traces if there is poor abdominal pick-up, or for monitoring the presenting fetus in multiple pregnancy. Their use is contraindicated where there may be a risk of vertical infection (HIV, HBV, HSV, etc.), a fetal bleeding diathesis and in severe prematurity (e.g. < 32–34 weeks).

Liquor assessment

> Meconium staining of the liquor is associated with an increased chance of fetal distress. A normal CTG provides reassurance, but an abnormal CTG becomes even more significant if meconium is present, and should lower the threshold for investigation or intervention.

As well as being a sign of fetal distress, meconium is found below the cords postnatally in about one-third of cases in which it is present, and may give rise to the meconium aspiration syndrome. Clinical features range from mild neonatal tachypnoea to severe respiratory compromise. The incidence is probably unrelated to pH (and indeed the majority of babies with meconium aspiration

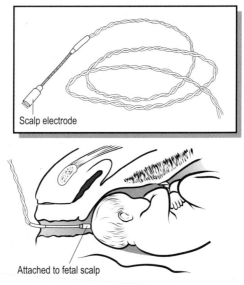

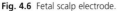

Fig. 4.6 Fetal scalp electrode.

syndrome are not acidotic at delivery), but the syndrome is more likely to be severe if there is associated acidosis. It is also more severe when the meconium is thick. There is no evidence to support early delivery as a prophylactic measure in the absence of fetal distress, as it is likely that the aspiration occurs in utero rather than at delivery itself. It is therefore accepted by many that routine suction on the perineum carries no benefit (and may cause apnoeas and bradycardias).

Fetal pH measurement

Fetal blood sampling is almost always used to establish further information following a suspicious CTG and perhaps to prevent unnecessary intervention. Consider alternatives. For example, if the head is well down at full dilatation, delivery might be more appropriate, as it would also be if the cervix is insufficiently dilated and the CTG is clearly highly suspicious (e.g. preterminal bradycardia). A pH of > 7.25 is normal, one of 7.20–7.25 is borderline (repeat in around 30 minutes unless the CTG improves) and an abnormal pH is < 7.20.

Association between CTG and pH

If all 4 components of the CTG are normal, the risk of a pH < 7.20 is ≈ 2%.

If 1 or 2 components of the CTG are abnormal, the risk of a pH < 7.20 is ≈ 20%.

If 3-4 components of the CTG are abnormal, the risk of a pH < 7.20 is ≈ 50%.

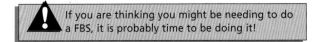

If you are thinking you might be needing to do a FBS, it is probably time to be doing it!

Place the mother in lithotomy with a 15° lateral tilt (or the left lateral position if approaching full dilatation). Insert an amnioscope appropriate for the dilatation and dry the scalp with a sponge or swab on long sponge-holders. Spray the scalp with ethyl chloride to induce hyperaemia and cover with a thin layer of paraffin jelly (so that the blood will form a blob and not run). Use the blade to make a small nick in the scalp and touch the blob with the capillary tube. Try not to touch the scalp directly (occludes the tube) and avoid admixture with any maternal blood in the vagina. Take three samples if possible to ensure consistency of results.

Fetal scalp pH correlates very poorly with Apgar scores. It is common practice to deliver if the pH is < 7.20.

- Only 15% of babies with pH < 7.1 have an Apgar score of < 7 at 5 minutes.
- Only 20% of babies with an Apgar score of < 7 at 5 minutes have a pH < 7.1 (Lancet 1982;i:494).

Long-term prognosis following 'fetal distress'

Of those babies with an Apgar score < 3 at 10 minutes, two-thirds die within 1 year. Of the survivors, 80% are normal. Neonatal encephalopathy is a better guide to long-term outlook than are Apgar scores:

- Grade 1. Hyperalert, decreased tone, jittery, dilated pupils: usually resolves in 24 hours.
- Grade 2. Lethargic, weak suck, fits: 15–27% chance of severe sequelae.
- Grade 3. Flaccid, no suck, no Moro reflex, prolonged fits: nearly 100% chance of severe sequelae.

The prognosis is generally good if the baby does not develop grade 3 encephalopathy, or if grade 2 encephalopathy lasts < 5 days. Further clinical evaluation may be available from EEG (the incidence of death or handicap is low if the EEG is normal or near normal), CT (the prognosis is good if the CT is normal or shows only patchy hypodensities) or USS (the incidence of impairment correlates with intracerebral hypoechogenic areas of necrosis). The incidence of cerebral palsy in term infants has not changed with 'improved' obstetric care, and probably < 10% of cases are due to intrapartum events (BMJ 1999:1054).

HAEMORRHAGE (SEE ALSO PV SPOTTING, P. 66)

> **This may be rapidly fatal. Beware of the tendency to underestimate the severity of the bleeding. Mobilize help from obstetricians, anaesthetists, midwives, the blood transfusion service, porters and senior haematologists. You cannot have enough help.**

> **⚠** Do not carry out an antenatal PV examination until placenta praevia has been excluded. No PV until no PP!

Antepartum haemorrhage

This is defined as PV bleeding at > 24 weeks and occurs in 3% of all pregnancies.

- Abruption.
- Placenta praevia (see p. 65). Placenta praevia caesarean sections should be supervised/performed by a senior obstetrician, especially when the placenta is anterior.
- Uterine rupture (see p. 109). This occurs only very rarely.
- Vasa praevia (beware when a succenturiate lobe is diagnosed). There is rapid fetal distress and usually no time for App's test.

Management

- Carry out maternal and fetal assessment, including an accurate calculation of the gestation, CTG and USS for the placental site.

- Consider delivery and the method of delivery (note there is an increased risk of PPH). Induction of labour is often relatively easy, although there is a small risk that the delay may exacerbate fetal distress and any coagulopathy.
- Gain IV access with two Grey Venflons. Take bloods for: Hb, H'CRIT, platelets, clotting and crossmatch RCC (the number of units depends on the volume lost).
- Give crystalloid or colloid (Haemaccel or Gelofusine, *not* Dextran) as required.
- See Further management of haemorrhage, below.

Postpartum haemorrhage

This is defined as > 500 ml blood. It is commoner in grand multiparity, multiple pregnancy, fibroids, praevia, following an APH and in those with a past history of PPH.

The PPH is *primary* if it occurs < 24 hours post-delivery. It is *secondary* if it occurs 24 hours to 6 weeks postdelivery.

Primary PPH is due to:

- in 90% of cases, atony ± retained products of conception
- in 7% of cases, trauma
- in 3% of cases, coagulation problem (usually DIC)
- multiple causes may be present.

Management

- Rub up a contraction by abdominal massage.
- Gain IV access with two Grey Venflons. Take bloods for Hb, H'CRIT, platelets, clotting and crossmatch RCC (the number of units depends on the volume lost).
- Give Syntocinon 10 IU stat. IV and then 20 IU in 500 ml Hartman's solution at 125 ml/h or faster if required.
- Give crystalloid or colloid (*not* Dextran) as required.
- Remove the placenta. Try continuous cord traction initially. If the placenta is retained, a regional block or GA will be required, but pethidine 50 mg IV with midazolam 2–10 mg IV may be used if necessary. If there is placenta accreta and there is no bleeding *do not attempt any further removal*, but leave and manage conservatively.
- Give further oxytocics, e.g. Syntocinon 20 IU slow IV, ergometrine 0.5 mg slow IV or carboprost (Hemabate) 250 µg (= 1 ml = 1 ampoule) IM or intramyometrial (*not* IV) with further doses not less than15 minutes apart. Hemabate is contraindicated with cardiac, pulmonary, renal or hepatic disease. Side-effects include GI upset, particularly diarrhoea, and pyrexia. Consider also misoprostol 800 µg PR.

- Under GA, check for vaginal or cervical lacerations with general or spinal analgesia ('walk the cervix' with Rampley's sponge-holding forceps). In unexplained PPH, laparotomy should not be unduly delayed.
- See Further management of haemorrhage, below.

Further management of haemorrhage (J Obstet Gynecol 2003:463)

- Consider a CVP if the clotting is normal.
- Transfuse, ideally with warmed blood under pressure (filtration not usually necessary). O-negative or group-specific uncrossmatched blood may be used if required. Each unit of RCC ≈ 260 ml. Give 10 ml of 10% calcium chloride (or gluconate) IV over 10 minutes for every 6 U of RCC (sodium citrate preservative binds calcium). Major transfusion may lead to hyperkalaemia.
- Correct the coagulation defects of DIC with:
  — FFP (usually in packs of 300 ml), which contains clotting factors.
  — Cryoprecipitate. This is prepared from FFP and is a rich source of fibrinogen, factor VIII and von Willebrand factor. Use if the fibrinogen is low.
  — Platelet concentrate (needs to be ABO and Rhesus compatible). This is stored at room temperature (do not refrigerate) and is generally only required if the platelets are $< 50 \times 10^9/l$ in the presence of active bleeding (note damaged transfused platelets may aggravate DIC).
  — There is no indication for tranxenamic acid (risk of fibrin deposition in kidneys) or aprotinin (may also have anticoagulation properties) in DIC.
- Conservative measures to arrest bleeding from an atonic uterus include:
  — Balloon tamponade with a Rusch balloon (BJOG 2001:372), Senstaken–Blakemore tube or foley catheter.
  — Uterine packing (e.g. with 5 m long, 4 inch wide gauze pack).
- Surgery may be required to control the bleeding. Consider a B-lynch suture (BJOG 1997;372) or a simpler modification (Curr Opin Obstet Gynecol 2001:127). Radiologically directed arterial embolization is potentially a very useful option if available.
- Ligation of the vessels supplying the uterus is technically difficult, especially in the presence of a pelvic haematoma. It involves identification and ligation of the anterior trunk of the internal iliac artery distal to the origin of the posterior branch. The peritoneum is opened and the ureter (which passes medially over the bifurcation

of the common iliac artery) retracted to allow mobilization of the internal iliac artery and identification of the posterior branch. Confirmation of the femoral pulse should be obtained prior to tying. Bilateral mass ligation is easier and safer. This involves placing a suture just above the reflected bladder flap or below the level of the caesarean incision and the suture should contain 2–3 cm of myometrium. A second suture medial to the ovary may also be of help.

- Hysterectomy (or subtotal hysterectomy) may eventually be required, especially if there is a non-lower-segment uterine rupture or placenta accreta.
- See also p. 132.

UTERINE RUPTURE

This may occur with obstructed labour in multiparous patients and with use of prostaglandins or Syntocinon. It virtually never occurs in primigravidae. It may also occur following previous caesarean section, particularly a classic section. The risk following a lower uterine segment caesarean, however, is low: for every 10 000 women attempting trial of labour there will be 27 additional symptomatic uterine ruptures, 1.4 perinatal deaths and 3.4 hysterectomies related to the rupture (BMJ 2004:19)

Symptoms and signs

Rupture may occur prelabour or in labour. When it occurs during labour:

- Classically, there is maternal tachycardia, shock, cessation of contractions, disappearance of the presenting part from the pelvis and fetal distress. Pain may be minimal or may be severe and there is variable PV bleeding (bleeding is intraperitoneal if there is a complete rupture) or haematuria.
- Rupture may present postpartum with a continued trickle of bleeding in the absence of another cause.

Management of antenatal rupture

- Set up an IV infusion.
- Crossmatch 6 U of RCC (see Haemorrhage, p. 106).

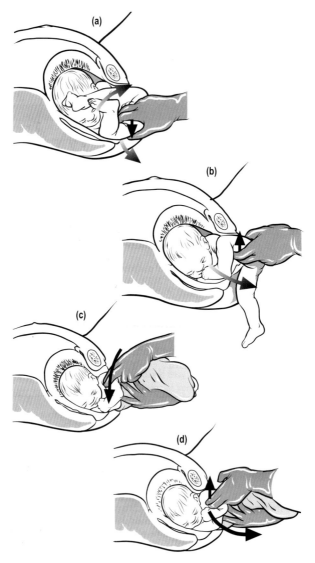

Fig. 4.8 (a) Flexion of left knee with a frank breech presenting left sacrotransverse. **(b)** Flexion of right knee. **(c)** Flexion of the left arm for **(d)** delivery under the symphysis pubis.

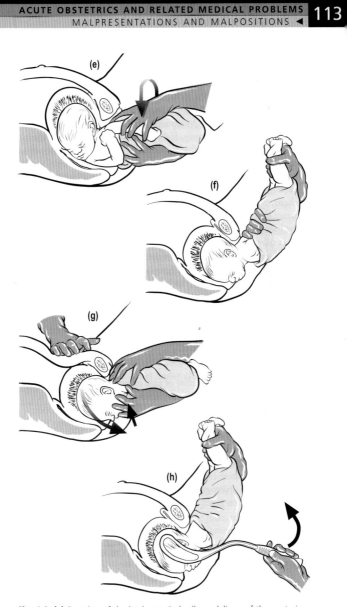

Fig. 4.8 (e) Rotation of the back anteriorly allows delivery of the posterior shoulder. **(f)** Lifting the body after allowing the breech to hang. **(g)** Mauriceau Smellie Veit for head delivery. **(h)** Alternative delivery of the head with forceps.

transverse incision above the bladder rather than risk unnecessary bladder trauma.

- Encourage the baby's head through the incision with firm, fundal pressure from the assistant (it may occasionally be helpful to use Wrigley's forceps). If the baby is breech, apply traction to the pelvis by placing a finger behind each flexed hip, or find an extended leg to pull and deliver with fundal pressure from the assistant. Encourage the assistant to 'follow' the head down, as this promotes flexion. If transverse, also try to find a leg (do not pull an arm).

After delivery, give Syntocinon 10 IU IV stat. and *wait for the uterus to contract* before delivering the placenta. Attain haemostasis with straight artery forceps. Check the uterus is empty and close with two layers of dissolving suture (e.g. Vicryl) to the uterus, one layer to the sheath and one layer to the skin. There is no need to close the peritoneum.

SHOULDER DYSTOCIA

> **Prompt, calm action is vital. Make the diagnosis after failure to deliver shoulders with the first downward pull of the head. The shoulders are stuck in the AP plane with the anterior shoulder behind the symphysis pubis.**

Management
Use 'HELPERR' (Table 4.4).
   If all else fails, the choices are:

- Try 'HELPERR' again.
- Fracture the clavicle (it may already be fractured after the above manoeuvres).
- Push the baby's head back up and perform a caesarean section (Zavanelli Manoeuvre).
- Perform a symphysiotomy:
   — Inject 10 ml of 1% lidocaine (lignocaine) plain to the skin over the symphysis pubis.
   — Do not abduct the legs > 80° (use two assistants to hold the legs).
   — Insert a foley catheter into the urethra, sliding it to one side out of the way with one hand.
   — Using the other hand, insert a scalpel under the skin, blade away from you, and make one stab incision approximately at the junction between the lower third and the upper two thirds of

TABLE 4.4 HELPERR mnemonic

H	Help	As with all obstetric emergencies the first response is to crash bleep the emergency team
E	Episiotomy	This allows room for imminent internal manoeuvres and reduces the frequency of vaginal lacerations.
L	Legs	Known as McRoberts manoeuvre. With one midwife to each leg, the mother's legs are flexed hard against her abdomen and at the same time abducted outwards. This straightens the sacrum relative to the lumbar vertebrae and rotates the symphysis towards the maternal head, allowing the baby's shoulder to pass under by continuous traction on its head. This manoeuvre may be successful in 40–60% of cases
P	Pressure	With the legs in the McRoberts position, suprapubic pressure is applied to push the anterior fetal shoulder (CPR style) downwards towards the fetal chest in an attempt to rotate the shoulder into the oblique and also to reduce the bisacromial diameter. This is used in conjunction with continuing head traction. If constant pressure fails, a rocking movement may be tried
E	Enter	Also known as the Woods screw manoeuvre. The attendant's hand enters the vagina. The middle and index fingers are placed on the posterior aspect of the anterior shoulder and an attempt is made to rotate the shoulder forward. If this fails, those fingers are kept static and the index and middle finger of the other hand are placed on to the anterior aspect of the posterior shoulder. Both sets of fingers are again used to attempt rotation. If this fails the reverse Woods screw manoeuvre is attempted. The fingers on the posterior shoulder are withdrawn completely. The fingers on the anterior shoulder slide down the fetal back to the posterior aspect of the posterior shoulder and rotation is attempted again
R	Remove the posterior arm	The hand of the operator is passed into the hollow of the sacrum, the fetal elbow identified, the forearm flexed and then delivered by sweeping it across the fetal chest and face. Fractures of the humerus are not uncommon with this manoeuvre
R	Roll over	It is possible to displace the anterior shoulder during the act of turning the mother over into the all fours position. If not, an attempt can be made to deliver the posterior shoulder first, i.e. the shoulder nearest the ceiling! It is possible to try all the above manoeuvres again in this new position

the symphysis. When the scalpel tip is just felt by the hand supporting the urethra, rotate the scalpel up towards the mother's head, thus dividing the upper two-thirds of the symphysis. Take the scalpel out, rotate 180°, reinsert and partially divide the lower third of the symphysis in a similar way.

Post delivery

Beware of PPH. Check the baby for asphyxia, brachial plexus injury, fractured clavicle and fractured ribs. The recurrence rate in subsequent pregnancies is probably around 15% (Am Journal Obstet Gynecol 2001:1427). It is unclear how to manage subsequent deliveries, but it is probably reasonable to aim for vaginal delivery in those who have had less severe shoulder dystocia, particularly if other deliveries have been without problems.

RETAINED PLACENTA

> **With oxytocics and continuous cord traction, 97% of third stages are complete by 10 minutes. The physiological third stage should be less than 30 minutes, but waiting until 60 minutes (rather than 30) halves the number of women requiring manual removal. Retained placenta is more likely if a previous manual removal has been required. There is an increased risk of PPH.**

Management

- Use continuous cord traction while protecting the fundus with the other hand to prevent uterine inversion.
- If not delivered:
  — Carry out a VE to ensure that the placenta is not sitting in the vagina. If nearly out, it may be possible to remove it with Entonox or midazolam 2–10 mg IV stat. (caution: respiratory depression, see p. 129).
  — If not, set up an IVI and crossmatch 2 U of RCC. Give prophylactic antibiotics (e.g. co-amoxiclav 1.2 g IV stat.).
  — Use a spinal or epidural block or GA for manual removal in theatre. If the placenta does not separate, it may be a placenta accreta. If not bleeding, do not attempt any further removal, but leave and manage conservatively. If the patient is bleeding, a hysterectomy may be required (see Haemorrhage, p. 106).
  — When the cavity is empty, give oxytocin 10 IU IV stat.

UTERINE INVERSION

> This is usually an iatrogenic problem. Suspect uterine inversion if there is profound shock without an obvious cause. The inversion may be partial or total.

Management

- Do not detach the placenta until the uterus is replaced and contracted.
- If the prolapse is easily reducible, try to reduce it.
- Start antishock measures with IV access and colloid.
- If reduction is unsuccessful, use hydrostatic reduction (O'Sullivan's): exclude perforation by clinical inspection. The inverted uterus is held within the vagina by the operator and the introitus sealed with the two hands of an assistant. Infuse 2 L of warm saline rapidly (e.g. with 1000 ml bags of saline through a silastic ventouse cup, urological Y giving set, or with a funnel and anaesthetic machine scavenging tubing).
- Once corrected, give Syntometrine 1 ml IM stat.
- If all this fails, consider laparotomy. It may be possible to partially divide the constriction ring, i.e. the ring formed at the point where the uterus has inverted. Hysterectomy may be necessary.

EPISIOTOMY REPAIR

See Figure 4.11.

POSTNATAL PROBLEMS

Puerperal pyrexia

This is defined as a temperature > 38°C on any occasion in the first 14 days after delivery or miscarriage (a slight fever is not uncommon in the first 24 hours). Pyrexia is usually due to urinary or genital infections (including endometritis), but may also be related to infection in the chest or breast. DVT and PTE must not be forgotten. After a full clinical examination (including breasts, legs, perineum and abdominal palpation of the uterus) send an MSU and endocervical ± wound swab for culture. If there is any suggestion of a chest infection, also send sputum for culture. Send blood cultures if the patient is systemically unwell.

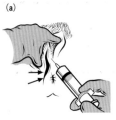
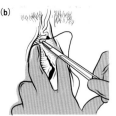
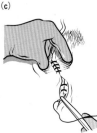
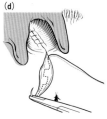
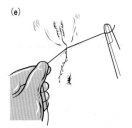

Fig. 4.11 Repair of episiotomy. **(a)** Infiltrate with 1% lidocaine (lignocaine) (unless epidural in situ or perineum infiltrated prior to delivery). Maximum lidocaine is 4 mg/kg (*NB: not 4 ml/kg*) without adrenaline and 8 mg/kg with adrenaline (e.g. 28 ml of 1% plain lidocaine in a 70 kg woman). Polyglycolic acid is the preferred suture material (*www.cochrane.co.uk 2004*), e.g. No. 1 gauge for the vagina and perineal body, and 2/0 for the skin. **(b)** Find the apex of the vaginal incision or tear and place the first suture above this level (*caution*: rectum posterior to vaginal wall). **(c)** Use a continuous locking suture to oppose the vaginal wall, continuing until the hymenal edges are opposed. The suture can then be tied or, more simply, locked, and the needle threaded between the opposed vaginal edges a few centimetres back ready to close the perineal body. **(d)** The perineal body sutures should be interrupted, and then a continuous finer suture used for the skin. It is possible that not closing the skin (i.e. leaving the skin edges approximately 5 mm apart) reduces postnatal pain. **(e)** Check instruments and swabs (a common cause of litigation in obstetrical and gynaecological practice). Carry out a PR to make sure that sutures have not penetrated the rectum.

> **Remember:**
> Carry out appropriate investigations if there is any
> suspicion of a venous thromboembolic disease (see
> p. 203).

In general, if the patient is well and the temperature only mildly
elevated, conservative treatment may be warranted. If the source of
infection is not clear, treat with either co-amoxiclav 2 tablets PO TID
(or 1.2 g IV TID) or with a combination of amoxicillin 500 mg QID
PO (or IV) and metronidazole 400 mg PO TID (500 mg IV). Treat
breast infections with flucloxacillin 500 mg PO QID. Breast-feeding
should continue.

Anaemia

This is common. It is reasonable simply to treat non-symptomatic
anaemia with oral iron, reserving transfusion for those with
troublesome symptomatology.

Breast problems

Two-thirds of women will have some problem, including nipple pain,
engorgement, cracks and bleeding. These can largely be prevented by
proper advice regarding positioning of the baby's mouth and
supportive counselling. Mastitis is frequently due to a blocked duct,
but can occur secondary to infection (e.g. *Staphylococcus aureus*, see
above). Breast-feeding should continue.

Superficial thrombophlebitis

This affects about 1% of women. There is a painful, erythematous and
tender (usually varicose) vein. Treat with support stockings and give
antiinflammatory drugs (e.g. ibuprofen 400 mg TID PO).

Secondary haemorrhage

This is defined as bleeding between 24 hours and 6 weeks postnatally.
It is usually due to infection or retained products of conception, rarely
to a vulval haematoma, very rarely to caesarean scar dehiscence and
only exceptionally to trophoblastic disease. Check P, BP, temperature,
uterine tenderness, haemoglobin and an endocervical swab. In
practice, the decision is usually between giving antibiotics or
arranging for an evacuation of retained products with antibiotic cover
under anaesthesia (this can often be done digitally, particularly in the
first week, without the need to instrument the uterus and risk
perforation). Clinical judgement is important, perhaps giving

antibiotics in the first instance if the bleeding is not severe, and arranging an evacuation if it does not settle. Do not rush into arranging an initial USS as many asymptomatic women have retained products after entirely normal deliveries and one is then tempted to carry out an unnecessary and potentially hazardous uterine evacuation.

Episiotomy breakdown

This is common, but long-term problems are rare. If the wound is clean, consider re-suturing. If there is any suggestion of infection, however, it is probably better to allow healing by secondary intention. Keep the perineum clean (e.g. baths or bidet BD) and consider antibiotics for infection.

The postnatal examination

This takes place at 6 weeks and should be a chance to review the delivery, answer any doubts or questions and place these in context for future deliveries. Also:

- How is the mother (tiredness, depression)?
- How is the baby?
- Check maternal Hb.
- Check cervical smear, if appropriate.
- Arrange contraception (see p. 213).
- Has intercourse been resumed? Any problems? (See p. 281).

ACUTE RELATED MEDICAL PROBLEMS

ACUTE PULMONARY OEDEMA

> **In obstetrics, the commonest cause is fluid overload, particularly in the presence of pre-eclampsia (see also ARDS, below).**

Management

- Identify and correct the underlying cause.
- Sit the patient upright and attach an O_2 saturation monitor, if available.
- Check ABGs and CXR.
- Give high-flow O_2 therapy.
- Give furosemide (frusemide) 50 mg bolus IV.

- Give morphine 5–10 mg bolus IV.
- A CVP line may assist with ongoing management, particularly in pre-eclampsia.
- Review drug therapy. Stop or avoid β-blockers (replace with hydralazine).

AMNIOTIC FLUID EMBOLISM

> This has a high maternal mortality (up to 80%) and is associated with multiparity, precipitate labour, uterine stimulation and caesarean section. Clinically there is sudden dyspnoea, fetal distress and hypotension followed within minutes by cardiorespiratory arrest ± seizures. It is often followed by haemorrhage from DIC and uterine atony, and may lead to ARF and ARDS. Differentiation from pulmonary embolism, anaphylaxis, aspiration, MI and abruption may initially be difficult. It is often diagnosed by exclusion.

Management

- Carry out CPR with high-flow O_2 ± IPPV and consider urgent delivery.
- Insert two large-bore IV lines and infuse with crystalloid or colloid, e.g. 2–4 units Haemaccel or Gelofusine until the BP is normal. Then stop the infusion to minimize the risk of ARDS.
- Check ABGs, U&E, LFT, FBC, clotting and crossmatch for 6 units of RCC.
- Correct any coagulopathy (see p. 108).
- As uterine atony is common, give oxytocics if delivered (see p. 107).
- Subsequent hypotension is usually due to cardiogenic shock; therefore consider transfer to the ITU for central monitoring ± a dopamine infusion.
- If a central line is used, send a sample of blood from the right side of the heart to the pathology department to look for 'squamous cells' to support the diagnosis (absence of squames does not exclude the diagnosis). Sputum should also be sent to look for squamous cells.
- See p. 133.

ANAPHYLAXIS

> An acute release of vasoactive substances leads to cyanosis, hypotension, wheezing, pallor, prostration and tachycardia.

Management

- Isolate the cause and remove (consider Latex allergy).
- Give high-flow O_2. If necessary, consider CPR or intubate for IPPV.
- Give adrenaline:
  — if severe, 5 ml 1:10 000 IM, or slow IV, or via an ET tube
  — if mild/moderate, 0.5 ml 1:1000 SC or IM, repeating in 10 minutes if required.
- Insert a large-bore (14 g) IV cannula and infuse 500–1000 ml colloid rapidly to re-expand the intravascular compartment.
- If wheeze is predominant, set up a salbutamol nebulizer 2.5 mg in 2.5 ml saline.
- Give hydrocortisone 100–200 mg IV over 2 minutes QID.
- Give chlorpheniramine 10 mg (i.e. 1 ml) IV over 1 minute.
- If there is deterioration, contact an anaesthetist.

MENDELSON'S SYNDROME

> This is due to inhalation of acid gastric contents. There is rapid onset of cyanosis, bronchospasm, tachycardia and pulmonary oedema. Differentiation from pulmonary embolus, congestive cardiac failure or amniotic fluid embolism may initially be difficult.

Prevention

- H_2 antagonist:
  — either ranitidine 150 mg PO 6 hours prior to operation;
  — or ranitidine 50 mg made up to 20 ml with normal saline IV given over 2 minutes closer to the operation.
- Sodium citrate 30 ml PO stat. prior to operation.
- Cricoid pressure with induction of GA.
- Aspirate gastric contents before waking from emergency GA.

Management

- Put the patient's head down and turn it to one side.
- Aspirate the pharynx and give 100% O_2.
- Give hydrocortisone 500 mg IV stat.
- Start ampicillin 500 mg QID IV and an aminoglycoside (e.g. gentamicin – give 4 mg/kg IV then daily at the same dose providing the gentamicin level 3 hours before the due dose is < 1 mg/l. If creatinine > 200 μmol/l, then dosage will need to be reduced).
- CXR, oximetry (or blood gases).
- Arrange physiotherapy.
- Later, bronchoscopy under GA and aspiration of mucus plugs may be of benefit.

CARDIORESPIRATORY ARREST

- If undelivered, consider lateral tilt.
- Commence basic and advanced cardiac life support (Fig. 4.12).
- Consider intrapartum causes (Tables 4.5, 4.6).

RESPIRATORY ARREST WITH OPIATES/ BENZODIAZEPINES/MgSO$_4$

Management

- Stop infusion of drug.
- Bag and mask with high-flow O_2, or intubate for IPPV.
- If *opiates*, give naloxone. This comes as 400 μg in 1 ml. Give 0.5 ml (200 μg) IV stat. then a further 0.25–0.5 ml (100–200 μg) as required.
- If *benzodiazepines*, give flumazenil. It comes as 5 ml of 100 μg/ml. Give 2 ml (200 μg) IV over 15 seconds, then 1 ml (100 μg) IV every 60 seconds to a maximum of 10 mls (1mg).
- If *MgSO$_4$*, see page 184.

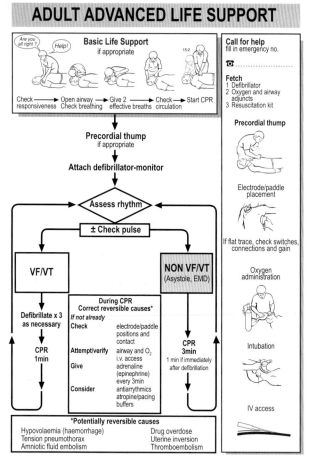

Fig. 4.12 Basic and advanced cardiac life support. (Based on the guidelines of the European Resuscitation Council, with permission.)

TABLE 4.5 Causes of sudden collapse

Cause	Features	Page
Amniotic fluid embolism	Is associated with multiparity, precipitate labour, uterine stimulation and caesarean section. There is *sudden dyspnoea, fetal distress* and *hypotension* followed within minutes by cardiorespiratory arrest ± seizures	127
Anaphylaxis	There may be *cyanosis, hypotension, wheezing, pallor,* prostration and tachycardia ± urticari	128
Cerebrovascular accident	May be past history of intracranial problems (e.g. previous subarachnoid haemorrhage). *Nausea and vomiting with headache*	175
Eclampsia	There is a *tonic–clonic seizure* (differentiate from epilepsy and amniotic fluid embolism from history)	183
Myocardial infarct	May be past history of heart disease. Chest pain	160
Tension pneumothorax	There is sudden onset of *pleuritic chest pain* (differentiate from pulmonary embolus) and diminished breath sounds	
Pulmonary embolism	There may be apprehension, *pleuritic chest pain, sudden dyspnoea, cough,* haemoptysis and collapse (differentiate from pneumothorax) ± antecedent risk factors	204
Uterine inversion	Occurs in the third stage only. It may lead to *profound hypotension* (There may be only a partial inversion and therefore the diagnosis may not be obvious	123

TABLE 4.6 Other emergencies

Other emergencies	Possible features	Page:
Asthma	Wheezing, use of accessory muscles, previous history	200
Haemorrhage	May be antepartum or postpartum. Bleeding may be underestimated, particularly in *concealed abruption* (hard painful uterus) or *uterine rupture* (shock, cessation of contractions, disappearance of presenting part from pelvis and fetal distress	106

SEPTICAEMIA

Septicaemia may rapidly kill. It is often caused by endotoxins from Gram-negative bacilli, but is also caused by anaerobes and exotoxins from aerobic and anaerobic streptococci. There may be dehydration, hypotension, cyanosis, pallor, cold extremities, hypothermia and jaundice. Multiple organ failure may ensue (see below).

Investigations

FBC (WCC > 15, platelets < 50×10^9/l), clotting screen (DIC), U&E, LFTs (?bilirubin) and ABGs (Pao$_2$). There may also be haemoglobinuria (following haemolysis).

Management

- Give high-flow O$_2$.
- Give IV colloid and consider a CVP line.
- Start antibiotics (blind):
  - gentamicin (see dose p. 129) (as bacteriocidal, endotoxins may lead to initial deterioration)
  - and metronidazole 500 mg TID IV
  - and ampicillin 500 mg QID IV.
- If there are retained products of conception, it is probably better to perform an ERPOC.
- If there is chorioamnionitis, deliver (vaginally or by caesarean section).
- A hysterectomy may have to be considered.
- Start heparin 5000 U BD or TID.

SYSTEMIC RESPONSE TO OBSTETRIC INSULT

Major haemorrhage or sepsis (and other triggers) may lead to multi-organ dysfunction syndrome (MODS). This may be related to the systemic inflammatory response syndrome (SIRS), a syndrome similar to that seen in sepsis, which leads to poor distribution of blood flow and a failure of cells to use oxygen because of the inflammatory process. SIRS is defined as two or more of pyrexia, tachycardia, tachyopnoea, raised white cells in response to infection, haemorrhagic shock or tissue injury (plus some other causes). (BMJ 1999:1606)

The systemic response may affect a number of different organs.

Lung

There may be increased pulmonary vascular permeability, which leads to alveolar oedema and refractory hypoxaemia (ARDS – Adult Respiratory Distress Syndrome). In obstetrics, it may also be secondary to aspiration, pre-eclampsia, or amniotic fluid embolism.

- *Stage 1*. There is hyperventilation with adequate arterial oxygenation.
- *Stage 2*. In the latent period, the respiratory rate is > 20/min and there are minor auscultatory changes of alveolar and interstitial oedema. There are also minor radiographic changes and hypoxaemia with a respiratory alkalosis. Treat with an O_2 mask and monitor with a pulse oximeter (aiming for > 90% saturation).
- *Stage 3*. There is respiratory failure refractory to high-flow O_2, usually occurring 24–72 hours after the initial onset of symptoms, with dyspnoea, tachypnoea, $\downarrow O_2$ and organization of hyaline membrane. There is bilateral diffuse infiltration on the CXR. Ventilate using positive peak end expiratory pressure ± central monitoring. There is no indication for prophylactic antibiotics per se, or mannitol.
- *Stage 4*. Irreversible shunting, severe refractory hypoxaemia and hypercapnia with metabolic and respiratory acidosis eventually lead to cardiac arrest.

Pitfalls of treatment

- Avoid fluid overload, especially with colloid.
- Invasive ITU monitoring with help from the anaesthetists is mandatory.
- High oxygen concentrations may contribute to further lung injury; therefore use the minimum O_2 concentration necessary to achieve > 90% saturation.

Heart

Myocardial dysfunction also complicates sepsis and the systemic inflammatory response syndrome. Ventricular dilatation occurs, and the ejection fraction may be reduced to around 30% despite an overall rise in measured cardiac output.

Kidney

Acute renal failure (ARF) is a common complication of sepsis and the systemic inflammatory response syndrome. The ability of patients to maintain intravascular homoeostasis may be impaired. ARF may also occur in obstetrics because of direct renal injury in pre-eclampsia, or bilateral ureteric injury. Acute renal failure is characterized initially by oliguria (usually < 400 ml in 24 hours) ± a rising creatinine and potassium, and may last days or weeks. There follows a polyuric phase, which may also last days or weeks (passing up to 10 l/day), and then finally, but not always, recovery.

The early use of haemofiltration to correct fluid imbalance and (possibly) remove circulating inflammatory mediators has been advocated, but the benefits are unproven. It is essential to restore circulating volume and achieve an adequate blood pressure and cardiac output to prevent and treat acute renal failure. Critically review all pharmacological agents and reduce doses accordingly (e.g. $MgSO_4$, aminoglycosides).

Bowel

The bowel is particularly susceptible to ischaemic insults. Hypoperfusion of the gastrointestinal tract is thought to be important in the pathogenesis of multiple organ failure as outlined above. Hepatic dysfunction, possibly resulting from reduced blood flow relative to metabolic demand, is also common in critically ill patients. Maintaining adequate flow and perfusion pressure are the only proven treatments to correct these deficiencies. Inotropic drugs with dilator properties such as dopexamine may selectively enhance splanchnic perfusion and oxygenation.

TRANSFUSION REACTIONS

> ⚠ It is essential to check that the name and number of blood products corresponds to that of the patient prior to transfusion.

Send all giving sets and bags to the BTS with 20 ml clotted blood. See Table 4.7.

TABLE 4.7 Transfusion reactions

Findings	Pathology	Management
Acute onset, becoming very unwell with fever and chills, shock, DIC, haemoglobinuria, oliguria, chest or back pains	ABO incompatibility → acute intravascular haemolysis (rare)	Stop the transfusion. Rx O$_2$. Support BP with normal saline or colloid. Take bloods: FBC, an EDTA for haptoglobulins (↑ in haemolysis), clotting (DIC), U&E (K$^+$ rises in haemolysis) and LFTs (including bilirubin). Also send 20 ml of clotted blood and an EDTA tube to BTS to confirm the diagnosis. ECG: risk of hyperkalaemia (see p. 170). Catheterize for hourly urine vols. Urine dipstix is usually positive for blood (haemoglobinuria). There is a risk of ARF (p. 133). Give furosemide (frusemide) 50 mg. If no diuresis, give 100 ml of 20% mannitol. If still no diuresis consider CVP monitoring and involve renal physicians. Also consider dopamine IVI 2–5 mg/kg/h. Repeat coagulation screens 2–4 hourly. Support with blood products if required (p. 108). If blood is still required, re-cross match. There is no increased risk of a second haemolytic reaction. See ARDS (p. 133) if appropriate

(Continued)

TABLE 4.7 Transfusion reactions (Continued)

Findings	Pathology	Management
Uncomfortable, but not unwell. May have fever and chills	Antibodies to leucocytes or platelets (common)	Slow or stop the transfusion Give antipyretics e.g. paracetamol 1 g PO QID Consider leucocyte poor red cells if recurrent
Acute onset of urticaria or rarely of anaphylaxis	Antibodies to plasma → allergic reaction (rare)	Stop the transfusion See 'Anaphylaxis' page 128 Give washed red blood cells if recurrent
Late onset (days) of fever, anaemia, hyperbilirubinaemia, but remaining relatively well	Non ABO, anti-RBC antibodies, e.g. Rhesus, Kell, Kidd, Duffy (rare)	Check the bilirubin level. Check a direct Coombs test Identify the antibody

CHAPTER 5

OBSTETRIC PRACTICE IN LESS DEVELOPED COUNTRIES

> Some practitioners who have lived, trained and worked in the
> UK decide to spend time in less developed countries, e.g.
> student electives, voluntary service or personal career choice.
> Clinical practice is likely to be very different from their
> previous experience and this chapter provides some guidance
> on how maternity care is delivered to the vast majority of the
> world's population.

INTRODUCTION

Maternity care in less developed countries is very heterogeneous: not
only are there wide variations between different countries, there is also
disparity in the provision of care between different parts of the same
country. While care in the urban private sector may be as good or even
better than that found in many developed countries, it may be
appallingly poor just a few miles away in a state-run health centre.

As it is impossible to generalize about the kind of patients one
would encounter and about the facilities that might be available, this
chapter will focus on what obstetric care is commonly like for an
underprivileged population: when resources are limited and
infrastructure back-up is scarce. It will also outline the basic
management principles at a peripheral health centre in a rural area and
finally mention the main problems that impact most on maternal and
fetal health in the developing world. The decision to attempt transfer
from a rural health centre to one with better facilities will always
depend on the patient's condition, the geography of the area, transport
and the patient's ability to pay.

Globally there are huge obstetric problems:

- Annually there are more than half a million maternal deaths
  worldwide: every minute, a woman dies from complications related
  to pregnancy and childbirth. Ninety nine percent of these deaths
  occur in the developing world.
- For every woman who dies during childbirth, around 20 more suffer
  injury, infection or disease.
- In some countries, 1 : 6 women have a lifetime risk of dying from
  complications related to pregnancy and childbirth. This compares
  with 1 : 2800 in the developed world (Table 5.1).
- One million children are left motherless each year due to maternal
  deaths: these children are 3 to 10 times more likely to die within
  2 years than children who live with both parents.
- The vast majority of maternal deaths are potentially preventable.

TABLE 5.1 Causes of maternal death

	Less developed countries	More developed countries
Maternal mortality rate	400 + /100 000 maternities	10 /100 000 maternities
Main causes:	Haemorrhage Indirect (malaria, anaemia, TB, HIV/AIDS, etc.) Sepsis Unsafe abortion Hypertensive disease Obstructed labour	Indirect (including suicide) Thromboembolism Hypertensive disease Sepsis Early pregnancy deaths Amniotic fluid embolism

CHALLENGES OF DELIVERING HEALTHCARE

Although scarce resources and poor infrastructure are predominant factors, there are also major social factors. The population may be diverse with low literacy levels, and with quite primitive beliefs and taboos. Furthermore, as some communities are isolated, outside interference in their local practices, however scientific and well meaning, may be seen with fear and scepticism. Geographical access can also be a major impediment to the uptake of medical services.

Try therefore to understand the local area, understand their practices, integrate with the health personnel at all levels, gain the confidence of local people and only then attempt to effect change. Learning the local language is, of course, a major advantage.

Blood

Blood is almost always in short supply, and therefore needs to be used extremely judiciously. Often it can be given only if a relative or a friend provides or replaces it and relatives will frequently refuse no matter how close and healthy the potential donor may be. 'I myself am the only earning member of the family, so what will happen if I donate and fall sick' or, from a mother-in-law, 'let her die; my son will get another wife but he won't donate blood' are examples of excuses. One may be able to purchase limited blood from the 'private' blood banks but since they frequently rely on paid donors, the chance of receiving unscreened blood with potential transmission of HIV or hepatitis B may be high. Conversely, unnecessary blood transfusions create risk from transfusion reactions and infection but most importantly use up an already scarce life-saving commodity.

Antibiotics

Antibiotic supplies are limited. Cheaper broad-spectrum oral antibiotics are generally available through state-funded health centres but IV antibiotics and other more expensive preparations (which may be needed for drug resistant strains) may not be available in remote locations, or will need to be purchased from outside the hospital. This will depend very much on the patient's ability to pay.

THE BASIC INFRASTRUCTURE

For many centuries, maternal and child health has been the preserve of untrained practitioners. Predominantly women, 'traditional birth attendants' (TBAs) have been, and still are, the mainstay of care provision in the rural parts of many countries. Until a few decades ago there was no formal training for TBAs and indeed some offered their experience as a community service or as a social responsibility. They learn the art of delivering babies from their elders and friends, and just continue this side-by-side with other regular occupations as farmers, domestics, etc. As they are a part of the local community they are often, not surprisingly, more trusted than formally trained professionals.

In the last few decades several countries have made efforts to incorporate the services of these practitioners into their national health schemes and have initiated formal training programmes. The main objectives of these programmes are to encourage mothers to attend for regular antenatal check-ups, receive iron and folic acid supplementation, identify pregnancy complications and refer to a more specialized centre if appropriate. They are also trained in safe and hygienic practices at the time of delivery, neonatal immunizations and records of births and deaths.

A comparative outline of the referral pathway is shown in Table 5.2.

In some areas, non-governmental and other charity organizations are the mainstay for provision of all aspects of healthcare including maternal and child health.

TABLE 5.2 A comparison of referral pathways	
Less developed area	*UK*
Traditional birth attendant (may be untrained)	
Medical officer – village health centre	GP/trained community midwife
District hospital/private hospital	District general hospital
Referral obstetric unit/private hospital	Tertiary level obstetric unit

The WHO uses the term 'essential obstetric care' to describe the elements needed for normal and complicated pregnancy, delivery and the postpartum period. Basic essential obstetric care services at the health centre should include at least the following:

- parenteral antibiotics
- parenteral oxytocic drugs
- parenteral sedatives for eclampsia
- facilities for manual removal of placenta and removal of retained products.

Comprehensive essential obstetric care services at the district hospital level should include the above plus:

- surgery
- anaesthesia
- blood transfusion.

Many peripheral centres do not adequately satisfy the above criteria.

APPROACH TO A PATIENT

> **Expect nothing and be prepared for anything! The work intensity may be light or the obstetric team might end up seeing more than 100 patients in one clinic.**

History taking

History taking has to be thorough but may need to be tailored according to the workload. With high levels of illiteracy, the history may be unreliable and there are often no formal case records. If you ask the right questions, though, the salient points are usually available. Remember that in many countries it is uncommon for unmarried women to be pregnant and in the antenatal clinic it is often assumed that the woman is married. Asking a pregnant woman whether she is married or not may incur the couple's wrath and create a scene you will almost certainly regret. If for some reason you need to clarify this issue, get a female nurse or helper in the clinic to do it for you.

Clinical examination

Be up to date with the basic clinical examination techniques and have a methodical approach to obstetric examination. In the absence of readily available investigations, you will be relying heavily on your clinical impressions. At some centres the only tools you will have to

Retained products of conception/puerperal sepsis

Retained products of conception/puerperal sepsis present with a combination of fever, abdominal pain and foul smelling vaginal discharge. In the absence of vaginal bleeding, it is reasonable to treat with IV antibiotics initially. If the patient has persistent vaginal bleeding then there is a strong possibility of retained products of conception, and an evacuation of the uterus may be required.

ENDEMIC CONDITIONS SEEN DURING PREGNANCY

ANAEMIA

Anaemia is common and results from a combination of malnutrition, frequent pregnancies, malaria and hookworm infections, and there is usually a microcytic, hypochromic iron deficient picture. Severe anaemia (Hb < 7 g/dl) is associated with low birth weight babies, increased perinatal mortality, cardiac failure and increased maternal mortality. Tests for malaria may be possible, but serum ferritin levels and folate assays are rarely available. Severe anaemia should always be treated (WHO recommends treatment when Hb < 10.5 g/dl). Treatment depends on the cause. Since iron deficiency is the most common cause, it is not uncommon to find most women attending the antenatal clinic on routine iron supplementation (ferrous sulphate 200 mg once or twice a day). If a woman has severe anaemia at term, the delivery should take place in an obstetric unit with facilities for close monitoring and blood transfusion.

MALARIA

In addition to being a significant cause of maternal death, malaria is also a major cause of perinatal mortality, low birth weight and maternal anaemia. There are estimated to be up to 200 000 newborn deaths/year in the malaria-endemic areas of Africa through *Plasmodium falciparum* alone. Person to person transmission occurs through the bite of a female Anopheles mosquito. Of the four types of human malaria, *Plasmodium vivax* and *P. falciparum* are the most common and *P. falciparum* is the most lethal. Malaria kills by infecting and destroying red blood cells (anaemia), and by clogging the capillaries that carry blood to the brain (cerebral malaria) and other organs. Typical symptoms include high-grade fever with rigors, headache, joint pains and, in the case of cerebral malaria, convulsions.

Malaria should be the first diagnosis considered in any pregnant woman presenting with fever in a malaria prone area. As convulsions may be misdiagnosed as eclampsia it is essential to treat the woman for both malaria and eclampsia until the diagnosis is confirmed. Pregnant women with severe malaria are particularly prone to hypoglycaemia, pulmonary oedema, anaemia and coma. The symptoms and complications will depend on the intensity of malaria transmission and the level of acquired immunity (higher immunity in areas of moderate or high transmission). A thick (blood) film will help detect the parasite and thin film will identify the species. If facilities for testing are not available, empirical treatment should be commenced.

Treatment depends on the local species prevalence and sensitivity profile. Chloroquine is considered safe in all three trimesters of pregnancy but chloroquine-resistant *P. falciparum* malaria is quite widespread. Quinine or a combination of sulphadoxine and pyrimethamine can be used throughout pregnancy to treat chloroquine-resistant *P. falciparum* malaria. Mefloquine, artesunate and artemether may be used in the second and third trimesters in pregnancy but there are limited data on their use in the first trimester. Antimalarials contraindicated for use during pregnancy are primaquine, tetracycline, doxycycline and halofantrine.

Treatment of uncomplicated malaria:

- Chloroquine-sensitive falciparum and *P. vivax* malaria: chloroquine 10 mg/kg body weight PO OD for 2 days followed by 5 mg/kg body weight for the third day of treatment.
- Chloroquine-resistant *P. falciparum* malaria: sulphadoxine/pyrimethamine 3 tablets PO as single dose (not to be used if patient is allergic to sulphonamides) or quinine salt 10 mg/kg body weight PO TID for 7 days.
- Chloroquine-resistant *P. vivax* malaria: sulphadoxine/pyrimethamine 3 tablets PO as single dose (not to be used if patient is allergic to sulphonamides) or quinine salt 10 mg/kg body weight PO BD for 7 days. Multidrug-resistant strains have been noted and management should be based on the national guidelines.

Treatment of complicated or severe malaria should ideally be at the level of a district hospital or above:

- Loading dose: infuse quinine dihydrochloride 20 mg/kg body weight in IV fluids (5% dextrose, normal saline or Ringer's lactate) over 4 hours (Never give an IV bolus injection of quinine).
- Maintenance dose: infuse quinine dihydrochloride 10 mg/kg body weight over 4 hours. Repeat every 8 hours (i.e. quinine infusion for

4 hours, no quinine for 4 hours, etc.) Continue this dose schedule until the woman is conscious and able to swallow and then give quinine 10 mg/kg body weight PO every 8 hours to complete 7 days of treatment.

- Monitor blood glucose levels for hypoglycaemia every hour while the woman is receiving IV quinine.

Prevention and control of malaria could have a major impact on maternal mortality. The strategies are:

1. Intermittent preventive treatment – involves providing all pregnant women with at least 2 treatment doses of an effective antimalarial drug during routine antenatal clinic visits. This approach is safe, inexpensive and effective (low birth weight babies reduced from 23% to 10% in one study).
2. Insecticide-treated nets decrease both the number of malaria cases and malaria death rates in pregnant women and their children.
3. Treat individual cases of malaria illness (who will then not transmit the infection).

HOOKWORM INFECTION

Two main organisms are responsible – *Ancylostoma duodenale* and *Necator americanus*. Infection may be asymptomatic but is a major cause of anaemia during pregnancy.

Treatment
Where the problem is endemic (prevalence of 20% or more), give one of the following treatments:

- albendazole 400 mg PO once or
- mebendazole 500 mg PO once or 100 mg BD for 3 days or
- levamisole 2.5 mg/kg body weight PO OD for 3 days or
- pyrantel 10 mg/kg body weight PO OD for 3 days.

Where the problem is highly endemic (prevalence of 50% or more), repeat the anthelmintic treatment 12 weeks after the first dose.

HIV/AIDS

Worldwide, about 40 million people are living with HIV infection and about half of all affected adults are female. Mother-to-child transmission (MTCT) is by far the most important cause of infection for the estimated over 5 million HIV-positive children. As noted on page 195, antenatal antiretroviral therapy reduces the chances of

MTCT but this is available to less than 10% of those infected. This proportion may increase with the '3 by 5' initiative (treat 3 million people by 2005, www.who.int).

The effectiveness of any programme to combat HIV/AIDS during pregnancy depends on the availability of HIV testing and counselling; the proportion of HIV infected women who are aware of their serostatus in pregnancy; the proportion of women seeking antenatal care; the quality of antenatal care; and ease and availability of drugs. HIV testing in pregnancy may have some benefits in terms of transmission prevention and care, but this must be balanced against the possible risks of stigmatization, discrimination and violence.

TUBERCULOSIS (TB)

Although an indirect cause of maternal mortality, TB is the biggest killer of young people and adults in the world today: it kills more women than all causes of maternal mortality put together. TB is also the leading cause of death in those affected by HIV/AIDS.

One-third of the world population is infected although only 10% of infected people have the disease. Pulmonary disease is the most common presentation, usually with cough, fever, weight loss, loss of appetite and haemoptysis. Diagnosis is made by examining three sputum samples under a microscope (CXR is more expensive and usually less accurate than sputum examination). Treatment involves multiple drugs most commonly rifampicin, isoniazid, ethambutol, pyrazinamide and streptomycin (all except streptomycin are considered safe in pregnancy and with breast-feeding). Short-course treatments run for 6–8 months and long-course treatments may run for up to 2 years, but multidrug-resistant strains have emerged. Consult the national guidelines and seek specialist advice if available. Since the treatment runs for several months, patient non-compliance is a major problem. DOTS (Directly Observed Treatment Short-course) is the only effective strategy in controlling TB on a mass scale (www.who.int).

Breast-feeding should be encouraged but if the mother is infective (i.e. sputum positive) postnatally, the baby should receive isoniazid prophylaxis and BCG vaccine.

OBSTRUCTED LABOUR

Obstructed labour is more common in the most deprived areas, but meticulous use of partographs can reduce the incidence. The most common cause is true cephalopelvic disproportion, but malpresentation is also important. Suspect obstruction if the woman has been labouring for more than 12 hours, particularly if she is short, malnourished, pyrexial, dehydrated and exhausted. There may be severe pain from a tonically contracted uterus or rarely because of uterine rupture. Abdominal palpation will often (but not always) reveal a tender and rigid abdomen and it may be difficult to identify the presentation; when it is possible, the presenting part is often deeply impacted in the pelvis: this may be more discernible on a vaginal examination (e.g. large caput and gross moulding in cephalic presentation). Fetal distress and intrauterine fetal death are common.

Plan for operative delivery. If the baby is alive then caesarean section should be performed; such operations can be challenging. If the fetus is dead, craniotomy and other destructive operations may be appropriate, but only by a very experienced operator. PPH, puerperal sepsis and urogenital fistulae are common.

UROGENITAL FISTULAE

Over 90% of urogenital fistulae in the developing world are of obstetric aetiology: an incidence of 1–2 per 1000 deliveries has been estimated worldwide. They result from prolonged compression of the anterior vaginal wall, urethra and bladder base between the fetal head and the symphysis pubis. In some parts of Africa, fistulae also occur from traditional surgical practices like female genital mutilation (www.amnesty.org). Vesico–vaginal fistulae are the most common but recto–vaginal and uretero–vaginal fistulae also occur.

Obstetric fistulae developing after obstructed labour should be treated initially by continuous bladder drainage, with antibiotics to limit tissue damage from infection (see also p. 308). Spontaneous closure of a urinary fistula can occur in 6–8 weeks with catheterization and conservative management. Prophylactic catheterization may also prevent a fistula formation after obstructed labour. Surgical management of these patients requires considerable expertise and specialist help is invaluable.

TETANUS

Neonatal tetanus is the most common form of tetanus in developing countries. It is caused by contamination of the umbilical stump with spores of *Clostridium tetani*. The contamination occurs following childbirth if the cord is cut with non-sterile instruments and/or because of traditional practices like applying animal dung to the cut cord. Tetanus may be seen in adults if the delivery has been conducted without proper aseptic precautions. Neonatal tetanus presents 3–14 days after birth. Classic symptoms are muscle spasms, initially of muscles of mastication causing 'lockjaw' and a characteristic facial expression – 'risus sardonicus'. This may be followed by a sustained spasm of back muscles – 'opisthotonus'. Later, even mild external stimuli may trigger generalized seizure-like activity leading to serious complications (e.g. dysphagia, aspiration pneumonia) that may prove fatal. Antitetanic serum and sedation are the basis of supportive treatment once symptoms develop. High dose intravenous penicillins are the antibiotics of choice.

Even with treatment, mortality can be high. Tetanus can be prevented by the use of tetanus toxoid. If given to the mother, antibodies cross the placenta providing immunity to the fetus against neonatal tetanus. For this purpose a woman should receive at least two doses of tetanus toxoid at least 4 weeks apart, with the last dose at least 2 weeks before delivery.

CONDUCT OF A NORMAL DELIVERY WITH MINIMAL SUPPORT

> **Remember the basics and do not panic: most babies deliver spontaneously without problems (p. 86).**

Ensure a warm room and use a partograph to manage the first stage of labour. In the second stage, maximize antisepsis as much as possible (e.g. wash hands often). If available use a delivery pack which usually contains a nail cleaning stick, a small piece of soap for cleaning the hands and perineum, a plastic sheet of about 1×1 m to provide a clean surface, a sterile razor blade, ties and gauze for the clean cutting and care of the umbilical cord.

If the woman has an urge to push in the second stage then allow her to push with uterine contractions; otherwise await further progress (if the second stage lasts for more than 2 hours without appreciable change then consider intervention or referral as appropriate). Check fetal heart rate at regular intervals and wait until the head is visible and perineum starts to distend. An episiotomy is recommended *only* if there is obvious perineal obstruction to the delivery of the head. Controlled delivery of the head is useful. Place one hand gently on the advancing fetal head and support the perineum with the other hand, covering the anus with gauze to prevent soiling. Ask the mother to breathe steadily and not to push during delivery of the head.

Once the head is delivered, feel for the cord. If the cord is around the neck then it may be slipped over the head or, if too tight, it may be clamped and cut. Await spontaneous rotation of the shoulders (usually happens in 1–2 minutes). Hold the baby's head and apply gentle downward pressure to deliver the anterior shoulder. Then lift the baby up towards the mother's abdomen to deliver the posterior shoulder. Note the time of delivery. Give the baby to the mother, clamp and cut the cord, dry the baby and assess breathing. If the baby's breathing is not satisfactory then commence resuscitation as below.

Assess uterine size to ensure that there is no second baby and then give oxytocin 10 IU IM to the mother. Monitor the condition of the uterus and check for vaginal bleeding. The signs of placental separation are lengthening of the cord and a gush of dark fresh blood. To deliver the placenta, place one hand just above the symphysis pubis to stabilize the uterus and with the other hand apply simultaneous gentle cord traction. *Do not apply excessive traction.* Check that the placenta is complete and check for vaginal tears. If placenta has not delivered 1 hour after delivery then commence an oxytocin 20 IU IV infusion over 2 hours and consider manual removal (p. 122).

NEWBORN CARE

> **Newborn care is complicated by traditional practices, at least some of which may be downright harmful but that are nonetheless deeply entrenched, e.g. applying animal dung to the cord stump, slapping the newborn to initiate breathing or immersing the baby in cold water. The basic needs of the newborn are warmth, cleanliness, breast-milk and vigilance. These may be most difficult to attain in the preterm. The 'Kangaroo Mother Care' initiative (*www.who.int*) is a useful way of caring for stable preterm and/or low birth weight babies by using uninterrupted adult body heat and exclusive breast-feeding.**

Basic resuscitation

Anticipate newborn breathing difficulties at certain births, e.g. prolonged and/or obstructed labour, fetal distress and/or meconium staining, prematurity and infection. Often, however, it is impossible to predict. A vigorous cry is a sign of a healthy baby and is also usually a sign that no further intervention is required. If there is no cry, then assess breathing and commence resuscitation:

- Check the airway – position the newborn so that the head is slightly extended. If there is meconium stained liquor, clear the airway by suctioning the mouth first and then the nose. This stimulus may sometimes be sufficient to initiate breathing. If spontaneous breathing does not start then
- Commence ventilation. Use an appropriate size mask to cover the infant's chin, mouth and nose. Squeeze the mask with two fingers and check for the rise of the chest. If the chest is not rising then recheck the airway (for blood or meconium obstruction), the head position or the seal between the mask and the face. Ventilate at about 40 breaths per minute. Continue ventilation until spontaneous cry/breathing is established. If breathing is slow (< 30 breaths per minute) or there is severe indrawing then continue ventilation and arrange transfer. The heart and lungs should be auscultated at regular intervals throughout ventilation.

Routine aspiration of the baby's mouth/nose/stomach, stimulation by slapping, tilting it upside down to clear the airways and unskilled intubation are ineffective, may actually be harmful, and should be strongly discouraged. If there is no response to ventilation after 20 minutes then resuscitation can usually be discontinued.

Thermal protection
To prevent hypothermia, ensure delivery in a warm room, dry the baby thoroughly, wrap it in a dry cloth and give it to the mother as soon as possible. The baby's mother is the best source of warmth! The baby may be bathed when the temperature is stable and the baby is doing well. Vernix has lubricating and anti-infection properties and does not need to be removed.

Cleanliness
Cleaning needs to be as meticulous as possible. It may be ensured by using a simple disposable delivery kit (see above). Keep the cord clean and dry and do not apply anything to it. No antiseptics are needed. If soiled, the cord can be washed with clean water and dried with clean cotton or gauze. If there are signs of infection, commence antibiotics.

Early and exclusive breast-feeding
Early and exclusive breast-feeding provides optimal nutrition. Breast-feeding should be started within the first hour of life, be on demand and exclusive (not even water). Use of bottles, teats and pacifiers should be discouraged. Traditional prelacteal feeds should be discouraged although harmless rituals may be allowed as long as they

do not delay breast-feeding. Early suckling provides colostrum which offers protection from infections and gives important nutrients. Exclusive breast-feeding reduces infant mortality due to common childhood illnesses such as diarrhoea and pneumonia. Frequent and exclusive breast-feeding is also an effective method of fertility regulation especially if suitable contraception is not available.

Eye care

Ophthalmia neonatorum is caused mainly by *Neisseria gonorrhoea* and *Chlamydia trachomatis*. In many countries, routine prophylaxis to prevent this is recommended. Silver nitrate 1% drops, tetracycline and erythromycin are all used topically but consult the respective national guidelines.

PRACTICES OF UNTRAINED/TRAINED BIRTH ATTENDANTS

Since a majority of births are attended by birth attendants, it is vital to become familiar with some of the local practices. These vary from region to region and a few examples are outlined below:

- During the antenatal period, herbal medicines and potions are administered – some may be beneficial. On the other hand some essential foods are withheld because of nutritional taboos.
- During labour the abdomen may be massaged in a certain way to change the position of the fetus.
- In obstructed labour, the abdomen may be pressed hard or forcefully massaged to aid the delivery of the baby. This is harmful and can lead to uterine rupture.
- In some societies obstructed labour is believed to be a punishment for marital infidelity.
- Postpartum haemorrhage is seen as cleansing the woman of 'bad blood' and may not be seen as dangerous!
- Maternal and fetal illness is at times attributed to evil spirits or bad omens, resulting in the delay or withholding of proper medical attention.

A few measures now considered to be old fashioned in the developed world but still practised in some areas: routine shaving, routine enema, routine episiotomy, keeping nil orally during labour, complete bed rest during labour and disallowing a birth companion. All these measures have been shown to be either ineffective or in some cases to cause more harm than good.

SUMMARY

The experience will undoubtedly be worthwhile and more than an eye-opener.

CHAPTER 6

MEDICAL DISORDERS IN PREGNANCY

Myocardial infarction

This is very rare in pregnancy but carries a high mortality, especially in the puerperium (25–50%). It may occur following coronary artery dissection in the absence of coronary atherosis. Troponin I is specific. Thrombolytic therapy is contraindicated during pregnancy as it may provoke placental haemorrhage. Those who have had an MI in pregnancy should be allowed to have a spontaneous delivery. A previous MI is not a complete contraindication to future pregnancies providing that cardiac function is satisfactory.

Cardiomyopathy

Puerperal cardiomyopathy This is rare (< 1 : 5000), carries a 25–50% mortality, and is associated with hypertension in pregnancy, multiple pregnancy, high multiparity and increased maternal age. It usually occurs in the puerperium (but may occur in late pregnancy) and presents with sudden onset of heart failure. There is a grossly dilated heart on echocardiography. Give furosemide (frusemide), nitrates, ACE inhibitors and digoxin. Heparin reduces the risk of thromboembolism. Deliver (ideally vaginally) if it occurs antenatally. If there is good initial recovery, the long-term prognosis is good (although there is a risk of recurrence in future pregnancies).

Hypertrophic cardiomyopathy This is relatively well tolerated in pregnancy unless there is severe outflow tract obstruction and heart failure. The risk of sudden death is probably not increased in pregnancy. Hypovolaemia should be avoided. Epidural anaesthesia should be used with caution only. Antiarrhythmic drugs may be required. β Blockers may be helpful in symptomatic patients.

Aortic dissection

Pregnancy is associated with an increased risk of aortic dissection, particularly in women with heritable connective tissue disorders (e.g. Marfan's syndrome, Ehlers–Danlos syndrome) or in those with aortic coarctation. Those with an aortic root diameter > 4 cm on ultrasound are at greatest risk, and risk may be increased further with hypertension ± a family history.

Dysryhthmias

Serious dysrhthymias are uncommon in pregnancy. Ventricular and atrial ectopic beats are common and are usually benign. Tachyarrhythmias are usually supraventricular. DC cardioversion, digoxin and adenosine are safe in pregnancy.

ENDOCARDITIS PROPHYLAXIS

This is required for those patients who have significant valvular heart disease and abnormal flow, those with prosthetic valves, and those who have had endocarditis. As treatment is simple, however, and the consequences of endocarditis grave, policies may vary in different areas:

- Give amoxycillin 1 g IV and gentamicin 1.5 mg/kg (not to exceed 120 mg) IV stat. Thereafter, give amoxycillin 500 mg IM QID (PO, IV or IM) 6 hourly until the baby is born.
- If allergic to penicillin, vancomycin 1 g by slow IV infusion (over 2 hours) with gentamicin 1.5 mg/kg (not to exceed 120 mg) IV may be more appropriate.

CONNECTIVE TISSUE DISEASE

ANTIPHOSPHOLIPID ANTIBODY SYNDROME

Lupus anticoagulant and antiphospholipid antibodies are associated with recurrent miscarriage, arterial and venous thrombosis, IUGR, pre-eclampsia and thrombocytopenia. Of women with a history of recurrent miscarriage (3 or more consecutive pregnancy losses), 15% have persistently positive results for phospholipid antibodies and have a rate of fetal loss of 90% when untreated. The diagnostic criteria for the antiphospholipid antibody syndrome are outlined in Table 6.1.

In those with APS who have a history of pregnancy morbidity (as defined in Table 6.1), there is evidence that low molecular weight heparin (e.g. enoxaparin 40 mg/day SC) together with aspirin 75 mg/day improves the outcome. Those with less than three miscarriages should be considered for aspirin 75 mg/day alone, to minimize the maternal risks of heparin exposure (thrombocytopenia, osteoporosis). In those with a history of thrombosis, it may be appropriate to increase the heparin dose midgestation (to, e.g. enoxaparin 40 mg bd). The lupus anticoagulant is present in around 30–40% of patients with SLE.

SYSTEMIC LUPUS ERYTHEMATOSUS (SLE)

SLE occurs in 1 : 700 women aged 15–64 years. It is more common in non-white populations. The diagnostic criteria are precisely set out, but essentially *four or more* of the following are required:

1. Malar (butterfly) rash
2. Discoid lupus
3. Photosensitivity
4. Oral or nasopharyngeal ulceration
5. Non-erosive arthritis involving two or more peripheral joints
6. Serositis (pleuritis or pericarditis)
7. Renal disorder (proteinuria > 0.5 mg/day, cellular casts)
8. Neurological disorder (seizures or psychosis)
9. Haematological disorder (haemolytic anaemia, leucopenia or thrombocytopenia)
10. Immunological disorder (Anti-DNA or lupus anticoagulant)
11. Antinuclear antibody.

TABLE 6.1 Antiphospholipid antibody syndrome (APS) is present if at least one of the clinical and one of the laboratory criteria are met

Clinical criteria	
Vascular thrombosis	Arterial or venous
Pregnancy morbidity	One or more unexplained death of a morphologically normal fetus > 10 weeks' gestation One or more preterm births < 34 weeks because of pre-eclampsia, eclampsia or severe placental insufficiency Three or more unexplained consecutive miscarriages < 10 weeks
Laboratory criteria	Anticardiolipin antibodies on more than one occasion at least 6 weeks apart Lupus anticoagulant on more than one occasion at least 6 weeks apart

Effect of pregnancy on SLE

There is probably no effect on the long-term prognosis (except in patients with pre-existing renal disease and impaired renal function) but there may be a slightly increased risk of flare up during pregnancy. Women should be strongly discouraged from becoming pregnant during disease flare-ups – active SLE nephritis during pregnancy is associated with a significant maternal and perinatal mortality and in particular with a risk of pre-eclampsia. Disease should optimally be in remission for 6 months before pregnancy.

Effect of SLE on pregnancy

SLE is associated with increased fetal loss rates from an increase in spontaneous miscarriage and preterm delivery. This is particularly so in those with raised anticardiolipin antibodies. Pre-eclampsia may be difficult to differentiate from a disease flare-up as both are associated with hypertension and proteinuria (look for low C3 and C4, urinary casts, high anti-DNA and evidence of SLE in other systems). The presence of blood in the urine, however, is more suggestive of SLE. There is no increase in the rate of structural fetal abnormalities, although there is a risk of fetal CHB in association with the presence of anti-Ro and anti-La antibodies. Neonatal lupus may rarely occur, and is characterized by haemolytic anaemia, leucopenia, thrombocytopenia, discoid skin lesions, pericarditis and CHB.

Management of SLE in pregnancy

- Check renal function with U&E and creatinine clearance.
- If lupus anticoagulant or anticardiolipin antibodies are present, commence aspirin 75 mg/day until 36 weeks' gestation.
- If there is a previous history of thromboembolic disease, or pregnancy morbidity, consider low-molecular-weight heparin throughout pregnancy (as for APS).
- If possible, maintain on simple analgesics (e.g. paracetamol) and try to avoid NSAIDs, particularly in the third trimester.
- Monitor disease activity with clinical assessment, urinalysis, complement levels (reduced in active disease) and anti-DNA (increased in active disease).
- Flare-ups should be managed where possible with oral prednisolone (if already on oral prednisolone prior to labour continue with hydrocortisone 200 mg QID IV in labour). Steroids should be reduced very cautiously in the puerperium because of the risk of further disease flares. If steroids fail to control disease, then azathioprine appears to be relatively safe. There are now good data to show that hydroxychloroquine does not cause fetal retinal damage. Methotrexate, cyclophosphamide and azathioprine should not be used during pregnancy and advice should be sought regarding discontinuation prior to conception.
- Regular growth scans should be carried out, looking for IUGR, as well as regular fetal monitoring with CTGs and biophysical profiles in the third trimester. There is no indication to deliver the fetus early unless there is evidence of fetal compromise, deteriorating maternal renal function or hypertension.
- CHB presents as prolonged fetal bradycardia on CTG and can lead to heart failure and non-immune hydrops. The baby may not cope with labour and CHB makes intrapartum fetal heart rate evaluation impossible. Elective caesarean section is appropriate.

RHEUMATOID ARTHRITIS

This usually improves during pregnancy although there is a risk of postpartum flare-up. There is no increased risk of fetal loss. There is, however, a small risk of CHB in association with anti-Ro or anti-La antibodies and there may be mechanical joint problems with delivery and anaesthesia. Treatment should be with simple paracetamol-based analgesics where possible. NSAIDs may be used with caution during the first and second trimesters but should be avoided if possible in the third trimester (where they are used, monitor the liquor volume). Prednisolone or occasional intramuscular or intra-articular depomedrone should be used to control severe disease if necessary. Sulphasalazine and hydroxychloroquine can be used but gold and penicillamine, methotrexate, leflunomide and anti-TNF therapies should be avoided both prior to conception and during pregnancy.

SCLERODERMA

Scleroderma even in its limited cutaneous form is associated with pulmonary hypertension in late disease; pre-pregnancy pulmonary function tests and an echocardiogram are appropriate. Hypertensive renal crisis may also occur in this form of disease, and careful attention should be given to monitoring of blood pressure and urinalysis. The diffuse cutaneous form, which is associated with internal organ involvement carries a poor prognosis for mother and fetus, and pregnancy should be discouraged.

DIABETES

- *Impaired glucose tolerance*: an abnormality of the oral glucose tolerance test without the threshold for the diagnosis of diabetes being reached.
- *Gestational diabetes*: carbohydrate intolerance that arises during pregnancy and disappears after delivery (therefore a retrospective diagnosis).
- *Established diabetes*: diabetes that existed before pregnancy.

Screening methods in pregnancy include the following (none is ideal):

- Random glucose measurements (do GTT if 7.0 mmol/l within 2 hours of meal or 5.5 mmol/l if after).

- GTT if obese, significant glycosuria, FH diabetes, previous babies > 90th centile, diabetes in a previous pregnancy or unexplained stillbirth.
- Oral GTT.
- Glycosylated Hb.

The normal fasting plasma glucose is < 5.5 mmol/l. For an oral GTT, patients should fast overnight. Venous blood is taken for fasting blood glucose and a 75 g glucose drink is given. Further venous blood samples are taken after 1 hour and 2 hours. The WHO non-pregnant criteria are:

- *Diabetes:* fasting glucose > 7.8 mmol/l and/or a 2-hour level of > 11 mmol/l.
- *Impaired GT:* fasting glucose ≤ 7.8 mmol/l and a 2-hour level of ≤ 11 mmol/l but ≥ 8 mmol/l. (*In pregnancy, a 2-hour glucose of ≥ 9 mmol/l and ≤ 11 mmol/l may be more appropriate.*)

The significance of impaired GT is controversial. It is associated with obesity and up to a half of those with impaired glucose tolerance in pregnancy go on to develop diabetes mellitus in the subsequent 25 years. There is no evidence that treatment is beneficial unless the results of the GTT suggest diabetes mellitus. It is reasonable to treat with diet in the first instance (unless the preprandial glucose is greater than 8 mmol/l) and to consider insulin if the preprandial level is still ≥ 6 mmol/l and/or the postprandial level is ≥ 8 mmol/l. The aim of insulin treatment is to keep the preprandial glucose level below 6 mmol/l.

Effects of pregnancy on diabetes

Insulin requirements may be static or decrease during the first trimester, increase during the second and third trimesters and may reduce slightly towards 40 weeks. Pregnancy exacerbates nephropathy, and in severe cases this may be an indication for termination. In poorly controlled diabetes, pregnancy may also exacerbate diabetic retinopathy and the eye should be monitored for proliferative retinopathy with laser treatment given if required. Ideally this should be pre-pregnancy. Paradoxically, visual acuity may deteriorate with better diabetic control.

Effects of diabetes on pregnancy

The incidence of pre-eclampsia is probably unchanged, but the risk to the fetus if this develops may be more severe. Polyhydramnios may result in unstable lie and malpresentation, and may also lead to preterm labour.

Effects of diabetes on the fetus and neonate

There is an increased risk of spontaneous miscarriage and the perinatal mortality rate is 2–4 times that of the normal population. The incidence of congenital abnormalities is also higher than in the non-diabetic population, perhaps several times higher, particularly cardiac defects, NTDs and renal anomalies. Caudal regression syndrome is very rare, but when it occurs it is almost pathognomonic of diabetes. The risk of congenital anomaly is increased if the maternal diabetic control is poor preconceptually and in the early stages of pregnancy, and also when there is evidence of maternal microvascular disease. Unexplained intrauterine fetal death (which is the other major contributor to perinatal mortality) may occur secondary to multiple factors, including chronic hypoxia, ketoacidosis, polycythaemia and lactic acidaemia. A macrosomic fetus may be more at risk because of the already increased oxygen demands.

Fetal macrosomia (> 90th centile) occurs in 25–40% of diabetic pregnancies. The risks are minimized if maternal blood glucose control prepregnancy is idealized and high postprandial blood glucose levels avoided. Labour and delivery may be complicated by dystocia and, in particular, shoulder dystocia. IUGR is associated with maternal vascular disease. Fetal hypertrophic cardiomyopathy, characterized by a thick intraventricular septum and left ventricular outflow obstruction, is more common in diabetic pregnancy and may cause fetal death. It is usually reversible over a few weeks if the infant survives. Neonates may have hypoglycaemia, hypocalcaemia, hypomagnesaemia and polycythaemia. There is also an increased incidence of respiratory distress syndrome as surfactant production is diminished.

Management of diabetes in pregnancy

At pre-pregnancy counselling advice should be given about good diabetic control, diet, smoking and folate supplements. Diagnose and treat retinopathy. Change those on oral hypoglycaemics to insulin. If possible, pregnancy management should be in a combined obstetric/diabetic clinic. Visits are often fortnightly. Blood glucose should be measured several times a day at home, aiming for tight control (e.g. with preprandial capillary levels < 5.5 mmol/l and 1–2 hour postprandial levels of < 7.5 mmol/l). HbA1 should be checked monthly. Insulin is commonly given in a soluble form preprandially three times daily, with a long-acting insulin overnight (a 'basal bolus regimen'). Ketoacidosis should be avoided, as it is associated with a significant perinatal mortality.

Maternal renal function, weight, BP and optic fundi should be checked at each visit. Offer serum screening and a detailed scan at

16–18 weeks to detect fetal anomalies. Examine the abdomen for polyhydramnios, macrosomia or IUGR (particularly common if microvascular disease is present) and consider serial growth scans. In the third trimester regular assessments of fetal well-being (Doppler, CTG or biophysical profile) may be carried out, but note that the CTG may be abnormal when plasma glucose is elevated or reduced. Also note that the use of liquor to assess fetal well-being may be flawed in diabetes as there is an increased possibility of polyhydramnios.

With regard to delivery, each case should be considered separately. There is no proven need for intervention before 40 weeks if there are no complications, and there is no indication for elective caesarean section on the basis of diabetes alone. If preterm labour occurs, steroids should be given as for the non-diabetic patient, but there may be marked deterioration in diabetic control (consider using an insulin IV infusion). β-Sympathomimetics may cause hyperglycaemia and should be avoided. The overall statistical chance of being delivered by caesarean section is around 50%, and there is around a 25% chance of having an instrumental delivery.

Contraception

The COC alters metabolism with a trend to worsening glucose tolerance and triglyceride levels. It may be the progestogenic component that is responsible for this, with an observed increased risk of thrombotic or thromboembolic events being related to the oestrogen components. The levonorgestrel-containing IUD may be better.

DIABETES AND DELIVERY

There are numerous different IV regimens. Some favour 'single infusions' (e.g. 10% dextrose with 10 mmol KCl and 10 U of Actrapid). An example of a 'separate infusion' regimen is outlined below. Always involve a diabetic physician.

It is important to differentiate those with IDDM from those with gestational diabetes. Those with IDDM will need insulin during delivery, whereas those with gestational diabetes, even if they have been on large doses of insulin during pregnancy, are unlikely to need insulin during labour and only rarely postpartum. It is most important to ensure that IDDM patients always have some insulin being infused. Discontinuing the infusion may result in ketosis within approximately 1–2 hours. In the immediate postpartum period most IDDM patients require no insulin, and regular glucose measurement is essential to re-establishing a subcutaneous regimen (the pre-pregnancy insulin requirement is a good starting point). Dextrose (5%) or normal saline may be used for IV fluid replacement. It is not necessary to use 5% dextrose solely; there is a risk of water overload and gluconeogenesis will continue in the fasting state anyway.

Caesarean section

This can be divided into six groups, as below.

Management

For those requiring insulin, make up an IV solution by adding 50 U short acting insulin to 50 ml of normal saline (1 ml = 1 U) and infuse according to the sliding scale in Table 6.2. Fluids can be given entirely independently of this.

IDDM patients undergoing elective caesarean section Give the normal insulin on the night before the operation (although consider reducing the intermediate or long-acting insulin). On the morning of the operation, omit the morning insulin, check U&E and glucose and insert an IV cannula. Infuse fluids and insulin as in Table 6.2.

Gestational diabetics who have required no insulin during pregnancy for elective caesarean section Perform glucose monitoring 4-hourly, although it is expected that all values will be < 10 mmol/l. Give IV fluids as required. If glucose levels are consistently above 10 mmol/l then commence insulin as above, stopping it on delivery of the placenta.

Gestational diabetics who have required insulin in pregnancy for elective caesarian section Give the usual evening insulin. Check the U&E and glucose on the morning of the operation and establish IV access. Monitor glucose 2-hourly and commence insulin as in Table 6.2 if the glucose is >10 mmol/l. Stop any infusion after the delivery.

TABLE 6.2 Sliding scale for insulin administration by IVI	
Glucose (mmol/l) every 2 hours	Rate of infusion (ml/h)
> 16	4
13–15.9	3
10–12.9	2
6.5–9.9	1
< 6.5	0.5

IDDM patients undergoing emergency caesarean section Check the U&E and glucose. Start an IV infusion of 5% dextrose 500 ml over 4 hours and run insulin through a separate infusion as in Table 6.2. Postdelivery insulin requirements frequently drop, so switch the infusion off and monitor the glucose every 2 hours. Recommence the infusion if the glucose is > 10 mmol/l. Continue IV fluids, adding potassium to the bags if required. Discontinue the insulin infusion 30 minutes after the first SC insulin injection to ensure an adequate overlap.

Gestational diabetics who have required no insulin during pregnancy undergoing emergency caesarean section No specific measures are required and insulin therapy is unlikely to be needed. Carry out glucose testing every 4 hours and commence an insulin infusion if > 10 mmol/l. IV fluids may be given as required. Stop any infusion after the delivery.

Gestational diabetics who have required insulin in pregnancy undergoing emergency caesarean section Check the preoperative U&E and glucose. Establish IV access and give dextrose 500 ml over 4 hours. Check glucose 2-hourly and give insulin if the glucose is > 10 mmol/l. Stop any infusion after the delivery.

Vaginal delivery
Management
For all those who have required insulin antenatally:

- It is possible to manage patients with their normal SC insulin and oral intake in labour, providing labour is progressing normally.
- If the patient needs to fast, commence an IV infusion with 500 ml 10% dextrose at a *constant* rate of 100 ml/h. Make up an IV solution of insulin as above (1 ml = 1U) and infuse according to the sliding scale in Table 6.2, checking the glucose on an hourly basis.
- Stop the infusion immediately postdelivery, continuing hourly glucose measurements for the first 4 hours. Recommence SC insulin (at previous non-pregnant dose) when the glucose is > 10 mmol/l.

DIABETIC KETOACIDOSIS

There is a high fetal loss rate due to fetal hypoxia from keto- and lactic acidosis. It occurs most commonly with IDDM, but may rarely occur with gestational diabetes, especially if β-agonists are used. The aim is to restore intravascular volume, lower the glucose, monitor electrolyte status and correct the acid–base balance.

Investigations

- Serum glucose and urinalysis for ketones.
- FBC, U&E, creatinine, glucose, ABGs and G&S.
- Fetal assessment with CTG and consideration of delivery depending on gestation and fetal well-being. Delivery of a compromised fetus should be delayed until the mother is metabolically stable. Correction of metabolic imbalance may reverse signs of fetal distress.
- Search for a cause: consider blood cultures, HVS, MSU and sputum for bacteriology, CXR, ECG.

Management

- Establish IV access and give 1000 ml of 0.9% saline and 6 U Actrapid IV stat. while awaiting the blood results.
- If Na^+ > 155 mmol/l, give 0.45% saline at 1000 ml/h until the Na^+ is < 155 mmol/l. If the Na^+ is < 155 mmol/l, continue with 0.9% saline at 125 ml/h for 4 hours.
- Set up a continuous insulin infusion (after stat. dose as above). Add 50 U of Actrapid to 50 ml normal saline and run it at 5 U/h until the glucose is < 14 mmol/l (increase to 10 U/h if the glucose is not < 25% in 2 hours). Thereafter give 500 ml of 10% dextrose with 10 mmol KCl in each bag at 100 ml/h and Actrapid as below:
  — if glucose > 12 mmol/l, add 14 U to each bag
  — if glucose 7–12 mmol/l, add 10 U to each bag
  — if glucose < 7 mmol/l, add 6 U to each bag.
- Add KCl to each bag depending on the K^+ result (5 ml of 15% KCl = 10 mmol), re-checking the level initially every 1–2 hours:
  — K^+ < 3.0 mmol/l, 40 mmol in each bag
  — K^+ 3.0–4.0 mmol/l, 20 mmol in each bag
  — K^+ 4.0–5.0 mmol/l, 10 mmol in each bag,
  — K^+ > 5.0 mmol/l, give no K^+.
- If > 6.5 mmol/l, there may be tented T waves with a prolonged QRS and there is a risk of arrhythmias. Give 50 ml of 50% dextrose IV and 10 U Actrapid IV. If > 8.0 mmol/l, also give 10 ml 10% calcium gluconate slow IV (for cardioprotective effect).
- If the pH is < 7.10 on ABG give 40 mmol (i.e. 40 ml) of 8.4% $NaHCO_3$ slow IV.

HYPOGLYCAEMIA

This is defined as blood glucose is < 2.2 mmol/l, although symptoms may occur before this level.

- If conscious, give sweet tea, milk, dextrose tablets or Hypostop.
- If unconscious:
  — 1 mg (1 vial) of glucagon IM or SC (should be available at home)
  — if no response, give 20–50 ml of 50% dextrose IV (irritates the vein)
  — if there is no glucagon and a vein cannot be found, give 50 ml of 50% dextrose via a nasogastric tube.
- Consider the cause.
- Do not omit the next dose of insulin.

DRUG MISUSE

> The prevalence of drug misuse is on the increase, particularly in women of childbearing age. Serious problem misuse is associated with socioeconomic deprivation, and an increase in obstetric complications including miscarriage, APH, IUGR, IUD and preterm labour. Care must usually be directed firmly towards social factors before any impact on obstetric problems can be achieved. Pregnancy may provide a window of opportunity to offer real help, breaking a cycle of poor parenting, which would lead in turn to further problems in the next generation.

History should cover the following:

- Type of drug:
  — street drugs (e.g. heroin, amphetamines)
  — pharmacological preparations (usually illicit and/or prescribed) e.g. benzodiazepines, buprenorphine and analgesics (particularly DF 118 and other codeine compounds)
  — prescribed preparations (usually methadone).
- Pattern of use, dose, route, frequency and method of financing supply.
- Social support, the other children, partner, family, friends, social work involvement, clothing, food, shelter and transport.
- Impending legal problems.
- Risks of infection, including HIV, hepatitis B/C counselling ± testing (see p. 193).
- Domestic abuse is a common occurrence with all groups of pregnant women, and all women should be asked about this (it is not any more common in association with socioeconomic

deprivation). Female drug misuse is often a consequence, rather than a cause, of violence.

- The woman may have poor self-esteem following a lack of trusting relationships, a lack of a positive body image and concerns about her own ability to be a parent.

Management

Social factors Illegal drugs are expensive and addicts are often forced into theft (and therefore problems with the police and courts) or prostitution (with its risks of violence and sexually transmitted diseases, including HIV). In addition, the lifestyle may be erratic and pregnancy outcome is compounded by various additional nutritional and social factors. Attendance for antenatal care may compete with more immediate problems (e.g. seeing the social worker, lawyer, or getting money/drugs), but if such care can be delivered locally with truly flexible access and be combined with confidentiality, non-judgmental consistency, access to social workers and legal aid, then fuller and more holistic care can be achieved.

Opiate/opioid users For these women, consider transfer to methadone (this is metabolized more slowly than opiates/opioids, and therefore remains at more stable levels: there is less risk of fetal distress and preterm labour associated with sudden withdrawals or fluctuations in serum opiate levels). Those stabilized on methadone alone probably have a lower neonatal mortality than those still taking heroin. There may also be improved prenatal attendance. There is still no appropriate substitution therapy for other commonly misused drugs.

Detoxification There are theoretical fetal risks from very rapid opiate/opioid detoxification, but in practice the true fetal risks from even 'cold turkey' detoxification are relatively small. It has been suggested that the risks of detoxification (whether rapid or gradual) may be higher in the first and third trimesters, but practical experience does not bear this out. The goal should be to reduce drug use to a level compatible with stability (e.g. with methadone), not necessarily aiming for abstinence. It may be more acceptable for a mother taking a moderate dose of methadone to top up with very small amounts of a similar non-infected substance (e.g. smoking heroin) rather than increasing methadone doses to very high levels in a futile attempt to achieve total abstinence from illicit drugs. In women who attempt unrealistic reductions in methadone and do top up with other drugs, the dose of methadone should be increased. Topping up with benzodiazepines is particularly inadvisable. Patients undergoing rapid detoxification should ideally be managed on an obstetric unit, or at least under the close supervision of an obstetrician.

Neonatal complications

The effects of 'recreational' drugs on the fetus are summarized in Table 6.3.

There is an increased incidence of low birthweight due to IUGR ± preterm delivery and SIDS. Opiate/opioid use is associated with an increased incidence of meconium aspiration. Withdrawal is particularly associated with opiates/opioids and benzodiazepines, and is worse if these drugs have been used together. Severity is dose

TABLE 6.3 Fetal effects of drugs	
Drug	*Effect on fetus*
Alcohol	There is no clear dose relationship. Fetal alcohol syndrome is rare (IUGR, microcephaly, craniofacial abnormalities and mental retardation). Consumption of even small amounts of alcohol has been associated with a reduction in birthweight and intellectual impairment
Amphetamines	There is no good evidence of fetal abnormality. Fetal thrombocytopenia is very rare
Benzodiazepines	Neonatal withdrawal occurs at levels associated with misuse, even after quite brief use
Ecstasy	No increased risk has been demonstrated
Cannabis (hash, marihuana)	There have been no demonstrable teratogenic effects, but there is an association with IUGR and possibly with preterm labour
Opiates/opioids (e.g. heroin, methadone, DF118, buprenorphine)	Methadone and heroin are associated with meconium staining and IUGR, and heroin is also associated with amenorrhoea (± anovulation) and preterm labour. Buprenorphine and DF118 probably have similar associations to heroin, but with DF118 there is increased severity of withdrawal
Cocaine and crack	Cocaine has been associated (rarely) with GU, limb/body and brain abnormalities (probably due to vasoconstrictive vascular accidents). There is an increased risk of abruption, PROM and possibly IUGR and SIDS
Nicotine	There is an association with IUGR, preterm labour, perinatal death and delayed development. Tobacco use, if heavy, may lead to neonatal withdrawals
LSD	There is a possible association with fetal abnormality

related and timing depends on the rate of drug metabolism (e.g. heroin and morphine are metabolized rapidly) and signs usually develop within 1 day, whereas methadone is metabolized more slowly and signs usually occur at 3–5 days. Babies are classically hungry, but feed ineffectually. There is CNS hyperexcitability (increased reflexes and tremor), GI dysfunction (finger sucking, regurgitation, diarrhoea) and respiratory distress. Treatment options include replacement (e.g. with methadone or Oramorph) for those who have been taking opiates/opioids. Replacement is not appropriate for benzodiazepine withdrawals. The severity of withdrawal symptoms is reduced by breast-feeding.

EPILEPSY AND OTHER NEUROLOGICAL DISORDERS

EPILEPSY

> Assume that a seizure during pregnancy is eclampsia until proven otherwise. Around a third of those with epilepsy have an increase in seizure frequency independent of the effects of medication, particularly those with secondary generalized or complex partial seizures. The fall in anticonvulsant levels due to dilution, reduced absorption, reduced compliance and increased drug metabolism is partially compensated for by reduced protein binding (and therefore an increase in the level of free drug). There is an increased incidence in fetal anomaly irrespective of the effects of drugs (3–4% vs 2% in the general population), possibly due to a combination of hypoxic and genetic factors. For those on anticonvulsants, the incidence of anomaly is at least 6%, and there is a possible later association with developmental delay and autism. Single-drug regimens are less teratogenic than multidrug therapy. Of the newer preparations, lamotrigine seems safe and may prove safer than the more traditional preparations.

Management
Pre-pregnancy counselling This is advised. Fertility is not impaired. Attempt to achieve seizure control with a single-drug regimen or, if seizure free for 2–3 years, consider drug withdrawal (this may have implications for the patient's work ± driving licence). Give preconception folate supplements 5 mg/day PO (anticonvulsants lead to a reduction in serum folate).

During pregnancy Continue folate supplementation until at least 12 weeks. Adjust anticonvulsant doses on clinical grounds (monitoring of plasma levels is usually not necessary, but can occasionally be useful to check compliance and exclude toxicity – 'free' drug levels rather than 'total' drug levels are ideal). If the level is low and the seizure frequency low, it may be acceptable not to increase the dose. In those taking anticonvulsants, it should be emphasized that there are fetal risks from the anticonvulsant medication as well as from not taking the drugs (from increased fit frequency). Offer aneuploidy screening as usual, but arrange a detailed fetal anomaly scan at 18–22 weeks (looking for neural tube, cardiac and craniofacial abnormalities as well as diaphragmatic herniae). For women on enzyme-inducing anticonvulsants (see below) give vitamin K 20 mg/day PO from 36 weeks (anticonvulsants are vitamin K antagonists and increase the risk of haemorrhagic disease of the newborn). The baby should be given vitamin K 1 mg IM stat. at birth and the paediatrician alerted to the possibilities of anticonvulsant drug withdrawal. Most fits in pregnancy will be self-limiting, but if prolonged, give Diazemuls 10 mg IV or diazepam 10 mg PR. If still continuing, give phenytoin by infusion and, if very prolonged, consider ventilation.

Postnatally The mother may breast-feed safely (drugs pass into the milk but are of little clinical significance). Advise about safe and suitable settings for feeding, bathing, etc. Carbamazepine, phenytoin, primidone and phenobarbitone induce liver enzymes, reducing the effectiveness of the standard dose COCs. Therefore, consider a 50 µg preparation (e.g. Ovran) or give $2 \times 25/30$ µg pills and reduce the number of pill-free intervals by running three packets together.

OTHER NEUROLOGICAL DISORDERS

Migraine

This generally improves in pregnancy. Paracetamol and antiemetics for treatment with β-blockers as prophylaxis are considered relatively safe. Focal migraine can occur.

Cerebrovascular disease

This is rare. Subarachnoid haemorrhage is nearly always secondary to an aneurysm (> 25 years old, > 30 weeks' pregnant) or AV malformation (< 25 years old, midtrimester or intrapartum). Those who have a previously clipped aneurysm should be allowed to labour, although it is reasonable not to allow a prolonged second stage.

Paraplegia

Assess renal function antenatally and check for urinary infection regularly. If the lesion is above T10, labour will be painless. If above T6, there is a risk of intrapartum autonomic hyperreflexia (leading to severe hypertension); therefore insert an epidural or give antihypertensives. Avoid bladder distension. Forceps are often required, caesarean section rarely so.

Multiple sclerosis

The risk of relapse during pregnancy is reduced, but is increased for 6 months postpartum, so that the overall relapse rate is the same as for the non-pregnant patient.

GASTROINTESTINAL DISORDERS

Peptic ulceration

Ulcers are rare in pregnancy but, when present, tend to improve. If ulcer symptoms occur, first-line treatment is with simple antacid/alginate compounds. If not resolving then use ranitidine 300 mg/day PO. Those with problematic recurrent ulcers should also take ranitidine. Endoscopy is the investigation of choice if necessary.

Inflammatory bowel disease (IBD)

Fetal loss rate is similar to that of the normal population, providing that the disease is not active at the start of pregnancy. Flare-ups of disease occur most commonly in the first trimester. There is no evidence of any fetal problems with prednisolone or sulfasalazine and these should be continued at the minimum dose necessary. Avoid constipation. Give folic acid supplements.

Acute episodes of IBD present with abdominal pain, diarrhoea and passage of blood and mucus PR. Patients should be admitted and the fluid and electrolyte balance checked. Stool samples should be sent for culture to exclude gastroenteritis. Treatment is with topical steroid enemas, oral sulfasalazine 1 g BD and prednisolone 10–20 mg/day. If the patient deteriorates, consider the possibility of intestinal perforation or toxic megacolon. Colostomies and ileostomies may become temporarily obstructed during pregnancy. Vaginal deliveries are preferable to caesarean section (as there is a risk of adhesions from previous surgery), although care is needed with operative vaginal deliveries if the disease involves the perineum. Although sulfasalazine crosses into breast milk, there is no evidence of any neonatal problems.

Coeliac disease

Presentation in pregnancy is rare, and the features are non-specific: GI symptoms, anaemia and weight loss. Antibodies to tTG, gliadin and endomesium are found in 90% with untreated disease (and they are relatively specific), but intestinal biopsy remains the gold standard for diagnosis (usually duodenal biopsy via endoscopy). Treat with a gluten-free diet and vitamin supplementation. Pre-pregnancy supplementation with folic acid is important to minimize the risk of neural tube defects, and patients should be encouraged to comply strictly with their gluten-free diet. The prognosis for the mother and fetus is good.

HEPATIC DISORDERS

A history of a prodromal illness, overseas travel or high-risk group for blood-borne illness may suggest viral hepatitis. Itch is suggestive of cholestasis. Abdominal pain is associated with gallstones, HELLP syndrome and acute fatty liver. Clinical signs are often unhelpful in diagnosis. Check the U&E, urate, LFTs, blood glucose, platelets and coagulation screen. Take blood for hepatitis serology. Upper abdominal USS may show obstruction or fat infiltration. Alkaline phosphatase increases in pregnancy (1.5–2 times normal).

LIVER DISORDERS SPECIFIC TO PREGNANCY

Hyperemesis gravidarum

If severe, this may be associated with abnormal LFTs (see p. 56).

Intrahepatic cholestasis of pregnancy

Incidence may be as high as 2% of pregnancies depending on definition and population, and it usually presents after 30 weeks' gestation. The main symptom is generalized pruritus, which may be particularly severe on the palms, soles and trunk, and which can be associated with anorexia, insomnia, steatorrhoea and dark urine. Symptoms usually disappear within 48 hours of delivery. It is likely that there is genetic predisposition to the cholestatic effect of oestrogens, with a positive family history in up to half of patients. There is a moderate (less than three-fold) increase in transaminases and a raised alkaline phosphatase (above normal pregnancy values).

Bilirubin is usually < 100 μmol/l. Serum total bile acid concentration is the most sensitive marker early in the disease.

There are no serious long-term maternal risks but there is a risk of preterm labour, fetal distress and intrauterine fetal death. The fetus must be monitored closely and delivery at 37–38 weeks is probably appropriate as tests do not accurately predict sudden death. Itch is difficult to control, but most will have improvement within 1–7 days of starting ursodeoxycholic acid at a dose of 8 mg/kg in divided doses (around 250 mg TID). This has not been shown to be beneficial (or harmful) to the fetus, but studies are too small to draw conclusions. It does, however, drop the level of bile acids. Give vitamin K 10 mg/day PO to the mother predelivery to minimize the risk of PPH. If LFTs do not return to normal after delivery, exclude primary biliary cirrhosis. The COC pill might also, but not inevitably, lead to pruritus and monitoring of LFTs is therefore prudent. Recurrence in subsequent pregnancies is high (45–70%) but not inevitable.

Overlap syndromes

Pre-eclampsia, eclampsia, HELLP syndrome and acute fatty liver of pregnancy are all pregnancy specific conditions. There is debate as to whether these are all part of a pre-eclampsia based spectrum or separate entities. The first three are discussed on page 181.

Acute fatty liver of pregnancy

Incidence around 1 : 10 000 pregnancies, although a trend towards identifying milder cases will increase this rate. This very rare condition carries a significant maternal mortality and fetal mortality (around 20% for both) and progression to hepatic failure may be rapid. There is an association with obesity, pre-eclampsia and male fetuses. It usually presents with vomiting in the third trimester associated with malaise, abdominal pain and fever. This is followed by jaundice, thirst and alteration in consciousness level. LFTs are elevated (AST ×3–10 normal), urate and neutrophils are high, and there is often profound hypoglycaemia. There is often also hypertension and proteinuria. Once the diagnosis is made, correct any coagulopathy, hypoglycaemia and fluid imbalance. Monitor the fetus continuously and prepare for delivery, usually by caesarean section. Following delivery there is a risk of PPH and liver dysfunction may be prolonged. Hepatic encephalopathy may develop and liver transplant is occasionally necessary. If the patient recovers, there is no long-term liver impairment. The recurrence for subsequent pregnancies is around 25%.

OTHER LIVER DISORDERS

Viral hepatitis

This is the commonest cause of abnormal LFTs in pregnancy. Check hepatitis A, B and C titres, as well as for CMV and toxoplasmosis (see p. 189).

Cholelithiasis

Asymptomatic gallstones do not require treatment. Cholecystitis should be managed conservatively with analgesia, bed rest, IV fluids and broad-spectrum IV antibiotics. Check amylase to exclude pancreatitis. Obstruction of the bile duct requires surgical treatment.

Cirrhosis

In severe disease there is usually amenorrhoea. If pregnancy occurs, and the disease is well compensated, there is usually no long-term effect on hepatic function. The main risk is from bleeding oesophageal varices. During pregnancy, patients should rest and take a high-carbohydrate, low-protein diet. Constipation should be avoided. Vaginal delivery is safe and usually appropriate. Sedative drugs should be used with caution as they may precipitate encephalopathy.

Chronic active hepatitis

This is usually associated with amenorrhoea. Pregnancy does not usually have any long-term effect on liver function. Obstetric complications are common and fetal loss rate is high. Immunosuppressant therapy with prednisolone and azathioprine should be continued in those with autoimmune disease.

Primary biliary cirrhosis

This is variable in severity. The prognosis for mother and fetus is good in mild disease. It may present during pregnancy for the first time in a similar way to intrahepatic cholestasis of pregnancy.

Acute pancreatitis

This may be more severe in pregnancy and the fetal loss rate is ≈10%. Serum amylase is markedly elevated. Treatment is with fasting, bed rest, IV fluids, oxygen and correction of any glucose and electrolyte balance (including calcium and magnesium).

HYPERTENSION

> Hypertension in pregnancy is defined as a diastolic BP
> > 110 mmHg on any one occasion or > 90 mmHg on two
> occasions ≥ 4 hours apart (ISSHP classification). Severe
> hypertension is a single diastolic BP > 120 mmHg on any one
> occasion or > 110 mmHg on two occasions ≥ 4 hours apart. In
> normal pregnancy the BP will fall during the first trimester,
> reaching a nadir in the second trimester and rise slightly
> again during the third trimester. Measure in the sitting
> position with an appropriate size of cuff. Although
> controversial, it is suggested that the phase IV Korotkoff
> sound (i.e. 'muffling' rather than 'disappearance') should be
> taken when reading the diastolic pressure.

Raised BP at booking (e.g. < 16 weeks) is usually due to chronic
hypertension (usually essential hypertension and only rarely renal
disease or phaeochromocytoma). Gestational hypertension and
pre-eclampsia (hypertension and proteinuria) only very rarely occur
< 20 weeks (with the exception of trophoblastic disease). Check FBC,
U&E and urine dipstix, and consider renal USS and separate 24-hour
urine collections for creatinine clearance and urinary catecholamines.

ESSENTIAL HYPERTENSION

This is commoner in older women and the prognosis overall is good.
The main risk is from superimposed pre-eclampsia (which is more
common with pre-existing essential hypertension). The hypertension
itself is rarely of significance, although there might be a slightly
increased risk of abruption. Those women, who are already taking
antihypertensive drugs, and who have mild to moderate hypertension
(140/90–170/110 mmHg), may be able to discontinue the medication
in pregnancy. Those with more severe hypertension should continue.

Treatment

Methyldopa This is the treatment of choice as it has a proven safety
record. An initial loading dose of 500–750 mg is appropriate, followed
by 250–750 mg QID PO.

β-blockers Labetalol can be used, but there may be an adverse effect
on fetal growth if used over a prolonged period of time (100 mg TID
to 400 mg QID PO).

Nifedipine This can also be used, and is particularly useful as a second-line agent where there is superimposed pre-eclampsia (10–30 mg PO up to QID).

Diuretics These should be avoided because of the relatively reduced intravascular fluid volume, particularly if there is any evidence of the development of pre-eclampsia.

ACE inhibitors These are contraindicated throughout pregnancy because of adverse effects on the fetal renal system, but are useful agents in the puerperium.

GESTATIONAL HYPERTENSION AND PRE-ECLAMPSIA

> - **Gestational hypertension: see definitions above, but note that some authorities also consider an incremental diastolic rise of > 25 mmHg above booking to be significant.**
> - **Gestational proteinuria:**
>   — **either ≥ 300 mg/24 h, or two clean-catch specimens at least 4 hours apart with ≥ ++ protein**
>   — **or ≥ + if the urine SG is < 1.030 (i.e. dilute) and the pH is < 8 (higher false positive rates with alkaline urine; overall false positive rate with dipstick ≈ 10%).**

Pre-eclampsia is a multisystem disorder of unknown aetiology peculiar to pregnancy and characterized by hypertension, proteinuria and, often, fluid retention. There is reduced maternal plasma volume and increased vascular permeability, some degree of intravascular coagulopathy (may lead to DIC), glomerular damage (proteinuria), liver dysfunction (see HELLP syndrome, p. 186), cardiac failure, pulmonary oedema, CNS problems (eclampsia, haemorrhage) and adverse fetal effects. It is an extremely variable and unpredictable condition, and progression is often more rapid the earlier in pregnancy it occurs. The purpose of antenatal screening is to prevent both the maternal complications (cerebral injury, multisystem failure) and fetal complications (IUGR, intrauterine death, abruption) of severe disease by timely delivery of the baby. Treatment of the mother with antihypertensives masks the sign of hypertension but does not alter the course of the disease; it may allow prolongation of the pregnancy and thereby improve fetal outcome.

Investigations

- Urate: this increases as pregnancy advances. Abnormal can be considered to be above 0.30, 0.35, 0.40 and 0.45 mmol/l at 28, 32, 36 and 40 weeks respectively.
- Platelets: these fall as the disease progresses, but should not be confused with the small physiological fall in platelets towards the end of pregnancy. The rate of fall of platelets is important as well as the absolute level itself.

Management of gestational hypertension
The following may be used as guidelines:

- If the BP is found to be elevated at an antenatal visit, recheck after 10–20 minutes. If settled, no further action is required.
- If the BP is elevated on ≥ 2 occasions ≥ 4 hours apart, appraise fetal size clinically, enquire about maternal well-being and advise to present if unwell or if frontal headache or epigastric pain (which can be severe). Check serum urate, U&E, FBC and platelets. Arrange twice-weekly BP recording and urine dipstix measurement.
- If there are abnormal blood results, or diastolic BP is > 100 mmHg, or has risen from booking by > 25 mmHg, or there is clinical suspicion of IUGR, or poor fetal or maternal well-being, arrange for a CTG and USS assessment of fetal size and liquor volume. Also, arrange BP recording and dipstix three times weekly, with at least weekly serum urate, U&E, FBC and platelets.

It is important to consider the overall picture rather than make decisions on the basis of a single factor. It is appropriate to admit the mother if there are symptoms or if there is significant proteinuria or severe hypertension. More intensive monitoring is possible, oral antihypertensives may be considered and plans can be made for delivery.

The decision to deliver and the method of delivery are dependent on many of the above factors and must be tailored to each individual patient. Conservative management < 34 weeks is associated with less RDS and necrotizing enterocolitis (*www.cochrane.co.uk* 2004) and is probably reasonable providing maternal BP, laboratory values and fetal parameters are stable. An epidural is probably contraindicated if platelets are < 100 × 10⁹/l (or ? < 50 × 10⁹/l). Ergometrine (including Syntometrine) should not be used for the third stage (give Syntocinon 10 U IM or IV stat. instead). It has been suggested that low-dose aspirin taken from early pregnancy (< 17 weeks and probably from the first trimester) may reduce the incidence of IUGR or perinatal

mortality in those with previous disease. Studies found that it may be
of benefit in high-risk situations and that it is safe (Lancet
1994;343:619). Haemorrhage is not a problem at this dose, even
though there is a moderate prolongation of bleeding time.

SEVERE PRE-ECLAMPSIA/ECLAMPSIA

Eclampsia is said to have occurred when there has been a convulsion.
The UK national incidence is 4.9/10 000 pregnancies, with 38%
occurring antepartum, 18% intrapartum and 44% postnatal. Of these
38% occur before proteinuria and hypertension have been
documented. The mortality is 1.8%, with a neonatal death rate of
34/1000 (BMJ 1994:1395). See the definition of severe hypertension
(above), but symptoms, or the presence of a coagulopathy, also
suggest severe disease.

Management of eclampsia

- Turn on side to avoid aortocaval compression.
- Insert an airway and give high-flow O_2 (e.g. 6 l/min).
- Give 4 g $MgSO_4$ IV over 10–15 minutes (details below).
- Consider urgent delivery if the fit has occurred antenatally.
- Set up a 1 g/h IV infusion of $MgSO_4$ (as below) and manage as for
  severe pre-eclampsia.
- Consider paralysis and ventilation if the fits are prolonged or
  recurrent.

Management of severe pre-eclampsia and ongoing eclampsia

The aim is to reduce diastolic BP to < 100 mmHg, prevent pulmonary
oedema, prevent convulsions and maintain the urine output.

- Gain initial IV access.
- Check the U&E, LFTs, albumin, urate, Hb, H'CRIT, platelets and
  clotting.
- Perform a CTG for fetal assessment.
- Give consideration to the method and timing of delivery.
- Catheterize.
- Measure hourly urine volumes.
- Control BP with hypotensive therapy.
- The aim is to reduce the BP slowly. Also consider giving labetolol,
  hydralazine (or nifedipine) as below.

Labetolol (Trandate) This comes as ampoules of 100 mg in 20 ml.
- Give an initial bolus: 50 mg (10 ml) slowly IV over 2–5 min.

- Then set up an infusion: add the ampoules undiluted to a syringe driver (5 mg/ml) starting at 4 ml/h, doubling every 30 minutes to a maximum of 32 ml/h (160 mg/h).

Side-effects. If used along with hydralazine there may be profound hypotension. Continuous BP monitoring is required and, if the patient becomes symptomatically hypotensive, give atropine 600 µg IV stat. Caution is required with asthma, and labetolol is contraindicated in those with AV block.

Hydralazine (Apresoline) This comes as ampoules containing 20 mg in powder form. Dissolve in 1 ml of water and make up to 20 ml with normal saline.

- Give a bolus: 5–10 mg slowly over at least 2 minutes.
- Then start an infusion: make this up as 80 µg/ml (i.e. 40 mg hydralazine to 500 ml Hartmann's solution). Start at 30 ml/h (40 µg/min), increasing by 30 ml/h every 30 minutes to 120 ml/h (160 µg/min) or until the BP is controlled. Wean off by reducing by 30 ml/h every 30 minutes.

Side-effects. Tachycardia and severe headache (therefore there may be confusion with eclamptic symptoms). Its use along with a β blocker may cause profound hypotension. Continuous BP monitoring is required, and if the patient becomes hypotensive give atropine 600 µg IV stat.

Nifedipine Give a 5–10 mg capsule sublingually, and repeat if required, to a maximum of 40 mg. (*Caution*: with $MgSO_4$, nifedipine may lead to increased BP.)
Side-effects. Headache (therefore it may be confused with eclamptic symptoms).

Anticonvulsant therapy

There is now very good evidence supporting the use of anticonvulsants in established eclampsia, and magnesium sulphate is known to be significantly more effective than phenytoin or diazepam in preventing further convulsions (Lancet 1995;345:1455). In those with severe pre-eclampsia, magnesium sulphate halves the risk of eclampsia and probably reduces the risk of maternal death (Lancet 2002;359:1877)

Magnesium sulphate (CI with myasthenia gravis)

- Take one 20 ml vial of 20% $MgSO_4$ (= 4 g) and infuse intravenously over 10–15 minutes. If the patient is anuric, do not administer further $MgSO_4$ until urine is produced. Providing there is urine production, infuse 1 g/h (5 ml/h) via a syringe pump, continuing for 24 hours after the last fit.

- If further convulsions occur, give a further 2 g (or 4 g if the body weight is > 70 kg) IV over 5 minutes.

Measure the respiratory rate and confirm that the patellar reflex is present (or forearm reflex in a patient with an epidural) every 15 minutes. If it is not possible to check these on such a frequent basis, $MgSO_4$ levels may be checked at 1 and 4 hours after commencement of treatment, and 6-hourly thereafter, aiming for 2.0–3.5 mmol/l. Although $MgSO_4$ is not sedative, it can depress neuromuscular transmission. Reduced patellar reflexes usually precede respiratory depression.

- If respiratory arrest occurs, intubate, ventilate, stop the infusion and give calcium gluconate (10 ml of 10% solution) over 10 minutes.
- If respiratory depression occurs, give high-flow O_2 (e.g. 6 l/min), stop the infusion and give calcium gluconate (10 ml of 10% solution) over 10 minutes.
- If the urine output is < 100 ml in 4 hours, reduce the $MgSO_4$ infusion to 0.5 g/h (2.5 ml/h) and review the fluid balance.
- If reflexes are absent, stop the infusion and restart it once reflexes have returned. Reduce the infusion rate (e.g. to 0.5 g/h = 2.5 ml/h) unless there have been further fits.
- If $MgSO_4$ is < 2.0 mmol/l, increase the infusion to 2 g/h for 2 hours and recheck.
- If $MgSO_4$ is 3.5–5.0 mmol/l, stop the infusion and restart at 0.5 g/h (2.5 ml/h), providing the urine output is > 20 ml/h. If $MgSO_4$ is > 5.0 mmol/l, manage as for absent reflexes.
- Continue for at least 24 hours postseizure.

Further management

- Involve senior obstetric and anaesthetic staff.
- Monitor the BP.
- Monitor the Sao_2. Consider measuring ABGs and arranging a CXR if the saturation drops below 93% or there is cough, dyspnoea or tachypnoea.
- Fluids given by IV infusion should probably not exceed 80 ml/h. Persistent oliguria (defined as < 30 ml/h) should prompt consideration of central monitoring. If fluid replacement is adequate and the plasma creatinine is < 100 mmol/l, there is probably no renal problem. If the creatinine is > 100 mmol/l, oliguria is probably due to abnormal kidney function, and infusions may cause pulmonary oedema. Anuria is always abnormal and may herald acute renal failure (see p. 133).

HELLP SYNDROME

HELLP is an acronym for haemolysis, elevated liver enzymes (particularly transaminases) and low platelets. It is probably a variant of pre-eclampsia, affecting 4–12% of those with pre-eclampsia/eclampsia, and is commoner in multigravidae. There may be epigastric pain, nausea, vomiting, and RUQ tenderness. AST rises first (> 48 IU/l) then LDH (> 164 IU/l). LDH > 600 IU/l indicates severe disease. A blood film may show burr cells and polychromasia consistent with haemolysis, although anaemia is uncommon. Platelet transfusion is rarely required with platelets > 40 × 10⁹/l, and is likely to be of benefit if < 20 × 10⁹/l and delivery is planned. There may be an increased incidence of abruption. There is also an increased incidence (although still rare) of hepatic haematoma and hepatic rupture, leading to profuse intraperitoneal bleeding. Management is to stabilize coagulation, assess fetal well-being and consider the need for delivery. It is generally considered that delivery is appropriate for moderately severe cases, but may be more conservative (with close monitoring) if mild. Postpartum vigilance is required for at least 48 hours. The incidence of recurrence in subsequent pregnancies is about 20%.

PHAEOCHROMOCYTOMA

This carries a high maternal mortality rate and may mimic pre-eclampsia. Hypertensive crises may be precipitated by anaesthesia or delivery (particularly caesarean section). Diagnosis is by 24-hour urine collection for catecholamines, and tumours should be localized with USS, CT or MRI scanning. Initial treatment is with combined α and β blockers such as phenoxybenzamine 20–40 mg/day PO initially, followed a few days later by propranolol 120–240 mg/day. Hypertensive crises may be treated with sodium nitroprusside. Surgical removal of the tumour can be performed before 24 weeks, but if diagnosed later in pregnancy is best delayed until fetal maturity when delivery can be performed by elective caesarean section at the same time as tumour removal.

INFECTION

It is often appropriate to seek bacteriological ± fetal medicine sub-specialist advice.

GENERAL

Farm workers

Toxoplasma (which causes miscarriage in cows and sheep), a chlamydia (which causes miscarriage in sheep), and listeria can all cause miscarriage in humans. Pregnant women should therefore avoid animal work, particularly in the lambing and calving seasons.

Basic hygiene precautions should be observed by all who are involved at this time. Overalls and boots worn for work should be removed at the house door, and the boots cleaned and left outside. Soiled overalls should be placed directly into the washing machine by the wearer, who should then wash and dry their hands thoroughly. At the end of the season the lambing/calving shed should be thoroughly washed and swept out, and left open to the air for the summer. Handwashing by all who enter the house from the farm at any time is the key to controlling such infection.

Food

- Soft cheeses: only soft cheeses made from pasteurized milk should be eaten, as there is a risk of listeria from unpasteurized milk and its products.
- Raw eggs: these must be avoided, as there is a risk of salmonella (remember puddings). Eggs need to be boiled for 8 minutes to kill salmonella reliably.
- Undercooked or raw meat or pâté may transmit toxoplasma, rarely listeria.
- Unwashed fruit: fruit should always be washed before eating as it may be contaminated with salmonella, toxoplasma or one of several intestinal parasites.

Nurses

Nurses may be concerned about CMV, particularly if they are in contact with small children. Serology is of little benefit, as the presence of antibodies does not necessarily denote immunity (see Table 6.4). Hands should be washed well and often. The risk of CMV is very small.

Travel and vaccinations

Consider aspirin ± graduated compression stockings for long-haul flights. If the woman is visiting a malarial region, give advice on mosquito nets, wearing long sleeves and trousers (tucked into socks), insect-repellent spray, cream, wipes, etc. Antimalarials should be taken (Lariam should be avoided if possible, although it may be safe > 12 weeks). The risk of vaccinations is likely to be small and probably outweighed by the risk of the disease.

There is an isolated thrombocytopenia without other haematological upset, splenomegaly or lymphadenopathy. Antiplatelet antibodies may be detected, but their absence does not exclude AITP. These antibodies may cross the placenta and cause fetal thrombocytopenia, although this is very rarely associated with long-term morbidity (unlike alloimmune thrombocytopenia – see below). No treatment is required in the absence of bleeding, providing the platelet count remains above $50 \times 10^9/l$.

Below this level treatment depends on clinical features. If there is bruising or petechiae, consider a short course of steroids (e.g. prednisolone 40 mg/day) or monomeric polyvalent human immunoglobulin (0.4–1 g/kg over 8 hours by IV infusion). If there is serious life-threatening mucous membrane bleeding, then platelet transfusion and urgent immunoglobulin is required. Avoid splenectomy in pregnancy. Platelets should be available in women with severe thrombocytopenia at delivery; there is little risk of bleeding from the placental site, but bleeding from incisions and lacerations may be marked.

In the absence of a history of ITP pre-dating pregnancy, and providing there are no detectable free IgG platelet antibodies, the risk of severe fetal thrombocytopenia is negligible. In view of this, it is difficult to justify pre-delivery transabdominal fetal blood sampling in all but the most selected cases, and there is a move towards much more conservative management. It is therefore very reasonable to aim for a vaginal delivery in most instances (and indeed there is no objective evidence that caesarean section is less traumatic). The only exception could be where the mother has entered pregnancy with pre-existing ITP and has currently identifiable PAIgG antibodies, or if treatment has been required during the pregnancy.

Other conditions

Thrombocytopenia may also occur with infection, drugs, alcohol, malignant infiltration of bone marrow, or be associated with megaloblastic anaemia, SLE (see p. 161) or HIV infection (see p. 195).

ALLOIMMUNE THROMBOCYTOPENIA

This is a rare disorder in which there are maternal antibodies to fetal platelets (much like the anti-red cell antibodies of fetal haemolytic disease). The maternal platelet level is normal, but there may be profound fetal thrombocytopenia, and antenatal or intrapartum intracranial bleeds. The diagnosis should be suspected when a previous child has had neonatal thrombocytopenia (usually associated with cerebral damage) and maternal antiplatelet antibodies have been identified (usually to the HPA-1a antigen). Treatment is controversial, but fetal platelet measurement by cordocentesis at 22 weeks has been used to assess the need for weekly maternal IV IgG (1 g/kg). This carries risks however and, although expensive, it is probably most appropriate to give maternal IV IgG regularly without performing any invasive fetal procedure. Some centres perform serial fetal platelet infusions, but there is a significant chance of procedure-related loss. Antenatal monitoring with USS may be appropriate, looking particularly for intracranial bleeding, and delivery should probably be by caesarean section for all. There is a 75–95% recurrence in subsequent pregnancies.

THROMBOEMBOLIC DISEASE

> **Normal pregnancy contributes to all three components of Virchow's triad. Venous thromboembolism is the commonest direct cause of maternal mortality in the UK (Confidential Enquiry into Maternal Deaths in the UK 2000–2002). The incidence of PTE is 0.3–1.2% of all pregnancies, with just over 40% of cases occurring antenatally, often in the first trimester. Over 80% of DVTs in pregnancy are left sided and > 70% are ileofemoral (unlike in non-pregnant patients). Risk factors include obesity, age > 35 years, high parity, previous thromboembolism, immobility, pre-eclampsia, varicose veins, congenital or acquired thrombophilia, intercurrent infection and caesarean section (particularly emergency caesarean section).**

Diagnosis of DVT

DVT may be asymptomatic; in addition to the traditional symptoms and signs, it may also present with lower abdominal pain. It is essential to make a definitive diagnosis if possible. Duplex Doppler ultrasound is particularly useful for identifying femoral vein thromboses, although iliac veins are less easily seen. This is safe and should be the first-line investigation. Venography is better, but has the disadvantage of radiation exposure and should be carried out if the Doppler scan gives equivocal results or is not available. Breast-feeding following contrast injection is safe. D-Dimer levels are slightly elevated in normal pregnancy.

Diagnosis of pulmonary embolism

(If collapsed, see Cardiorespiratory arrest, p. 129.)

Pleuritic chest pain, breathlessness, cough and haemoptysis are the major symptoms. These may be mild or there may be collapse and cardiopulmonary arrest. The ECG is frequently normal and the CXR is usually normal but may show a raised hemidiaphragm, atelectasis, reduced vascular markings, effusions or infiltrates. ABGs may show hyperventilation ($PCO_2 < 4.5$ kPa) and decreased O_2 exchange (e.g. $PO_2 < 8$ kPa). A VQ scan is required. Pregnancy is not a contraindication to this investigation and the risks are far outweighed by the benefits of diagnosis. A normal scan makes pulmonary embolism unlikely. A CT scan of the pulmonary artery may also be helpful.

Management of DVT or pulmonary embolism

Start treatment as soon as clinical suspicion arises; do not wait for a definitive diagnosis. Check a baseline coagulation screen and platelets. Instead of traditional heparin 5000 IU IV stat followed by a 1000 IU/h IV infusion with checking of the APTT after 6 hours and adjusting the infusion rate to keep the APTT 1.5–2 times the control, it may be reasonable to use low-molecular-weight heparin (Table 6.5), aiming for an anti-Xa level of 0.60–1.0 four hours after the injection. Anticoagulation should be continued until at least 3–6 months after the VTE event and for at least 6 weeks post partum. Treatment with streptokinase or caval filters may be useful in certain circumstances. Once anticoagulants are stopped, women should be screened for thrombophilia.

It is thought preferable not to be fully anticoagulated during labour. The options are to:

- Stop LMWH as soon as labour begins (though effects may last > 24 hours).
- Reduce doses to prophylactic level injections (e.g. enoxaparin 40 mg OD) prior to a planned induction of labour.
- Convert from LMWH to unfractionated heparin as more easily reversed.

Postnatally the patient may wish to continue with SC heparin or start warfarin 10 mg PO on days 3 and 4, adjusting the dose thereafter to keep the INR at 2–2.5 and stopping the heparin once the INR is stable. Warfarin does not cross into breastmilk in significant quantities.

Management of those with a previous thromboembolic history

Women who have had a single episode of DVT/PTE should be screened for thrombophilia. This can only be carried out

TABLE 6.5 Antenatal prophylactic and therapeutic doses of low molecular weight heparin (Reproduced with permission from RCOG, 2004)

Prophylaxis	Enoxaparin (100 units/mg)	Dalteparin	Tinzaparin[b]
Normal body weight (50–90 kg)	40 mg daily	5000 units daily	4500 units daily
Body weight < 50 kg	20 mg daily	2500 units daily	3500 units daily
Body weight > 90 kg[a]	40 mg 12-hourly	5000 units 12-hourly	4500 units 12-hourly
Higher prophylactic dose	40 mg 12-hourly	5000 units 12-hourly	4500 units 12-hourly
Therapeutic dose	1 mg/kg 12-hourly	90 units/kg 12-hourly	90 units/kg 12-hourly

[a]Body mass index > 30 in early pregnancy
[b]The dosage schedules for tinzaparin differ from the manufacturer's recommendation of once-daily dosage

comprehensively distant from the clotting event and after stopping anticoagulant medication. Check for the congenital thrombophilias, including antithrombin, protein C and protein S deficiency, the factor V Leiden mutation, the prothrombin gene variant, hyperhomocystinaemia and the antiphospholipid syndrome (see p. 161), which may be associated with an increased risk of fetal loss (those homozygous for the factor V Leiden mutation may also have a less optimum fetal outcome). If the screen is negative, and the event occurred outside pregnancy and was not severe, antenatal thromboprophylaxis may not be required. If the event occurred during pregnancy and the thrombophilia screen is negative then prophylaxis during pregnancy may be considered as below, and should probably be given postpartum.

Those who have had multiple thromboembolic events should commence antenatal prophylaxis, as below, 4–6 weeks in advance of the gestation at which their previous episode occurred, or sooner if additional risk factors, and continue postpartum. Those with a known congenital thrombophilia and previous venous thromboembolic event should probably also have prophylaxis antenatally and they should certainly have postnatal prophylaxis. This may also apply to women with a single episode of DVT/PTE together with a positive family history, even if the thrombophilia screen is negative. Patients with lupus anticoagulant or anticardiolipin antibodies should probably receive postpartum prophylaxis, and if they have a previous history of DVT/PTE, they should probably receive antenatal prophylaxis as well.

Antenatal prophylaxis Low-molecular-weight heparin (Table 6.5) SC once daily probably carries less osteoporosis risk than unfractionated heparin. The aim is to keep the antifactor Xa activity between 0.35–0.65 IU/ml. Platelet counts should be checked regularly because of the risk of heparin-induced thrombocytopenia.

Postnatal prophylaxis Heparin can be used as above. The patient may prefer to change to warfarin 2–3 days after delivery (heparin should be continued until the INR is 2–2.5). Treat for 6–12 weeks.

Risks of antenatal prophylaxis
Patients already on warfarin before pregnancy should be reviewed and should be changed to SC heparin. (The specific teratogenic risk of warfarin treatment in the first trimester is uncertain. Although the miscarriage rate is relatively high ($\approx$ 30%), the incidence of skeletal abnormalities, optic abnormalities and mental retardation is probably lower than was previously thought. There is also a risk of fetal intracerebral haemorrhage in later pregnancy. Warfarin is safe during breast-feeding). The only exception to this change is those with prosthetic heart valves: specialist advice should be sought.

Those who have a significant risk of thromboembolism should not be denied prophylaxis. Heparin may be associated with maternal thrombocytopenia and platelet counts should be monitored regularly during treatment. Long-term heparin therapy is also associated with maternal osteoporosis (fracture risk 1–2%). Heparin does not cross the placenta.

Remember
Warfarin may be reversed in the acute situation with 2–4 U of FFP IV stat. Heparin may be reversed with protamine sulphate 1 mg/100 U to a maximum of 50 mg (10–15 mg usually suffices).

Postnatal risk assessment

> ⚠ If you have performed a caesarean section or instrumental delivery, it is your duty to prescribe thromboprophylaxis.

The risks of thromboembolism should be assessed in all patients following caesarean section. Those at low risk should be mobilized early and receive appropriate hydration. Those at moderate risk (i.e. one or more risk factor, see Table 6.6) should receive unfractionated heparin 5000 IU SC BD for 5 days or until mobile.

It is also essential to consider prophylaxis in those who have had vaginal deliveries, whether instrumental or not.

TABLE 6.6 Thromboprophylaxis criteria

Low risk: early mobilization and hydration

Elective caesarean section – uncomplicated pregnancy and no other risk factors

---

Moderate risk: heparin (e.g. heparin 5000 U BD or enoxaparin 20 mg) and TED stockings

Age > 35 years

Obesity (> 80 kg)

Para 4 or more

Gross varicose veins

Current infection

Pre-eclampsia

Immobility prior to surgery (> 4 days)

Major current illness, e.g. heart or lung disease cancer; inflammatory bowel disease; nephrotic syndrome

Emergency caesarean section in labour

High risk: heparin (e.g. heparin 5000 U TID or enoxaparin 40 mg) and TED stockings

A patient with 3 or more moderate risk factors from above

Extended major pelvic or abdominal surgery, e.g. caesarean hysterectomy

Patients with a personal or family history of deep vein thrombosis; pulmonary embolism or thrombophilia; paralysis of lower limbs

Patients with antiphospholipid antibody (cardiolipin antibody or lupus anticoagulant)

THYROID DISORDERS

> In the Western world 1% of pregnant women are affected by thyroid disease, with hypothyroidism being commoner than hyperthyroidism. The fetal thyroid gland is active and secretes thyroid hormones from the 12th week. It is independent of maternal control, although maternal thyroid hormones do cross the placenta.

Measure:

- Free T_4 (normal range: 11–23 pmol/l in the first and second trimesters, 7–15 pmol/l in the third trimester).
- Free T_3 (normal range 4–8.5 pmol/l in first and second trimesters, 3–5 pmol/l in the third trimester).
- TSH (normal range 0.3–5.0 mU/l).

Hypothyroidism

This may present with fatigue, hair loss, dry skin, abnormal weight gain, poor appetite, cold intolerance, bradycardia and delayed tendon reflexes. If untreated there is double the rate of spontaneous miscarriage and stillbirth compared to the normal population, as well as a risk of fetal neurological impairment. There is minimal fetal risk if the mother is euthyroid.

In general, a low free T_4 concentration should be the impetus to increase thyroxine treatment rather than a raised TSH as the latter may remain elevated for a while after the free T_4 has returned to the normal range. (A raised TSH and normal free T_4 can also suggest non-compliance.) It is reasonable to monitor levels 8–12 weekly in those previously stable, but 4–6 weekly if adjustments are being made. Contrary to popular belief, the dose does not usually need to be increased in pregnancy. Fetal hypothyroidism may occur when the mother carries antithyroid antibodies or is receiving antithyroid drugs.

Hyperthyroidism

This presents with weight loss, exophthalmos, tachycardia and restlessness. It is usually due to Graves' disease, but may occur secondary to toxic thyroid adenoma or multinodular goitre. Untreated thyrotoxicosis is associated with significant fetal mortality and a risk of maternal thyroid crisis at delivery. Well-controlled hyperthyroidism is not associated with an increase in fetal anomalies. Graves' disease usually improves during pregnancy. It is worth noting that hCG has some thyroid stimulating activity and pregnancy (particularly molar pregnancy) may result in biochemical hyperthyroidism with normal or low TSH levels. If there are no clinical features of thyrotoxicosis, however, treatment is not required.

Optimal preconceptual control is ideal. In terms of the oral preparations there is little to choose between carbimazole and propylthiouracil; although they both cross the placenta, fetal thyroid suppression is rarely significant. The dose should be adjusted to keep the free T_4 at the upper range of normal, providing the patient is euthyroid, thereby minimizing the dose required. It is reasonable to check TFTs 4–6 weekly, unless adjustments are being made. Radioactive iodine is absolutely contraindicated, and surgery is indicated only for those with very large goitre, those with poor oral compliance and when malignancy is suspected. It may also be worth carrying out ultrasound growth measurements in case of IUGR. Neonates should be examined for goitre and cord T_4 and TSH checked.

Thyroid crisis

This is rare, but may occur in association with stress (e.g. labour) and presents with fever, tachycardia, atrial fibrillation, psychosis and coma. It carries a 10% mortality rate. Treat with propylthiouracil 1000 mg PO stat. initially followed by 200 mg QID (which can be given by nasogastric tube if necessary). One hour after the first dose, give potassium iodide 500 mg IV infusion TID (or orally QID). If there is no evidence of heart failure, give propranolol 0.5 mg IV stat. followed by 0.5 mg/min IV infusion or 80 mg TID PO. Chlorpromazine 25–50 mg 8-hourly PO or IV will treat psychosis and have a hypothermic effect. Rehydrate with IV fluids (e.g. dextrose) and treat heart failure with digoxin and diuretics.

Postpartum thyroiditis

This occurs following 5–10% of all pregnancies, with initial hyperthyroidism (low technetium uptake, unlike in Graves' disease) followed by hypothyroidism (around 1–3 months, therefore do not confuse with depression) and then recovery. Symptoms of hyperthyroidism may be treated with propranolol (antithyroid drugs accelerate the appearance of hypothyroidism). Treat hypothyroidism with thyroxine as above, withdrawing around 6 months postnatally. A small proportion may require long-term treatment or may develop hypothyroidism later in life.

CHAPTER 7

GYNAECOLOGY

ACUTE AND CHRONIC PELVIC PAIN

Symptoms, clinical findings and laparoscopic findings correlate poorly and ≈ 50% of those who are laparoscoped show no abnormality. Of those with pelvic pain, ≈ 50% show significant emotional disturbance, but studies have also shown that pain itself may lead to emotional problems. Some women will have un-voiced concerns about past relationships, and others will be concerned about implications of the pain for future fertility. A sympathetic and sensitive approach is essential.

Investigations

Symptoms suggest acute pain Consider the possible causes (Table 7.1), perform a pregnancy test, send vaginal swabs for infection (see p. 249) and arrange a pelvic USS. If investigations are negative and the patient is improving, adopt a conservative approach. If becoming worse, consider laparoscopy.

Symptoms suggest chronic pain Consider the above causes and investigations. Also consider laparoscopy and treat significant pathology if identified.

After laparoscopy (if no abnormality is identified) Reassure and review again in the outpatient clinic (if discharged without follow-up many will return with continuing pain). If the pain is still present, re-explore the history from the beginning. Listen, ask 'open-ended' non-directional questions, and try and discover the concerns and priorities of the patient. Consider using the label of 'chronic pelvic pain syndrome' as a disease entity in its own right and then devise strategies to relieve the physical, psychological and social distress that this causes.

Management options range from psychosocial, analgesia management, hormonal treatments and complementary therapies. Encouragement to lead as normal a life as possible while treatment is instigated is also acknowledged to be very important in the likelihood of making a full recovery. Complementary therapies such as reflexology, homeopathy and acupuncture may be helpful and should be encouraged if they are available and the patient is willing to pursue these alternatives. Refer to a psychologist if there is a high somatization score or history of sexual abuse.

TABLE 7.1 Causes of pelvic pain

Gynaecological	Gastrointestinal	Urinary tract
Ectopic pregnancy/ miscarriage	Appendicitis	Recurrent or chronic infection
PID (p. 249)	Constipation	Calculus (ureteric, bladder)
Ovarian cysts (especially torsion)	Diverticular disease	
Endometriosis (p. 237)	Irritable bowel syndrome	
Fibroids (p. 239)		
Adhesions		
Idiopathic		

Consider a 3-month trial of ovarian suppression. The COC may help, but may not suppress ovarian function completely. GnRH agonists are an effective, if expensive, treatment option. Provera 30 mg/day can also be used. A *dramatic* reduction of symptoms following ovarian suppression suggests a gynaecological cause. TAH and BSO is likely to be successful in improving pain in around 80% if suppression has been successful.

CONTRACEPTION

> The 'failure rate' in the absence of any contraception (i.e. the fecundity rate) is 80–90 : 100 woman-years. A summary of options is outlined in Tables 7.2 and 7.3.

NATURAL METHODS

During the fertile period cervical mucus is clear, watery (i.e. of low viscosity) and is easily stretched into strands (Spinnbarkeit). In the non-fertile period it is viscous. This knowledge, used in combination with a midcycle core temperature rise (0.5–1°C) and awareness that the fertile period is 6 days before to 2 days after ovulation, has a failure rate in *well-motivated couples* of 2.8 : 100 woman-years. Full unsupplemented breast-feeding in which the mother is amenorrheoic is 98% effective in the first 6 months. Another method should be introduced if menses occur (bleeding before 56 days following delivery can be ignored), or with the introduction of supplementary foods, or after 6 months.

TABLE 7.2 Principal side effects, dangers and risks of death of selected contraceptive methods

Method	Side-effects	Serious dangers	Risk of death	Failure rate per 100 women-years
Spermicides	Vaginal and urinary tract infections, allergy	None	None measurable	1.0–15
Cervical cap, diaphragm, sponge	Vaginal and urinary tract infections	Toxic shock syndrome	None measurable	
Condoms (male latex)	None	Anaphylactic reaction	None measurable	4.0–5.5
Combined oral contraceptives	Nausea, weight gain, dizziness, spotting, breast tenderness, chloasma, decreased libido	Cardiovascular complications, depression, hepatic adenomas, possible increased risk of breast and cervical cancers	Non-smokers aged < 35:1/200 000 Non smokers aged 35 + :1/28 600 Heavy smokers < 35: 1/5 300 Heavy smokers 35 + : 1/700	0.1–1.0
Progestogen-only oral contraceptives	Headaches, irregular bleeding, androgenic effects		None measurable	0.3–3.0
Emergency contraception (hormonal)	Nausea, vomiting, headaches, breast tenderness	None	None measurable	

(Continued)

TABLE 7.2 Principal side effects, dangers and risks of death of selected contraceptive methods (Continued)

Method	Side-effects	Serious dangers	Risk of death	Failure rate per 100 women-years
Injectables	Cycle changes, weight gain, headaches, changes in lipid profile, breast tenderness, post-discontinuation amenorrhoea	Depression, allergic reaction, possible bone loss	None measurable	0.1–1.2
IUD (copper)	Increased menstrual cramping, spotting and bleeding	PID following insertion, uterine perforation, iron deficiency anaemic	1:10 000 000	0.5–2.0
IUD (progestogen)	Initially may have increased menstrual problems; later reduced or even amenorrhoea. Spotting common.	PID following insertion, uterine perforation	1:10 000 000	<0.5
Implants	Tenderness at implant site, cycle changes, alopecia, weight gain, breast tenderness	Infection at implant site, depression, removal complications	None measurable	0.04
Female sterilization	Pain at incision site, possible regret that method is permanent	Infection at surgical site, anaesthesia complications, ectopic pregnancy	Laparoscopic tubal ligation: 1/38 500	0.15
Male sterilization	Pain at incision site, possible regret that method is permanent	Infection at surgical site, anaesthesia complications	Vasectomy: 1/1 000 000	0.04

LMP, Last menstrual period; PID, pelvic inflammatory disease.

TABLE 7.3 Medical eligibility criteria for selected family planning methods (World Health Organization)

Condition	Combined oral	Combined injectable	Progestogen only oral	Depot progestogens	Subdermal implants	Copper IUD	Levonorgestrel IUD
Age < 20	1	1	1	1–2	1	2	2
Age ≥ 40	2	2	1	1–2	1	1	1
Smoking	2–4	2–3	1	1	1	1	1
Obesity	2	2	1	2	2	1	2
Breast-feeding from weeks postpartum	2–3	2–4	1	1	1	1	1
Multiple risk factors for arterial cardiovascular disease	3–4	3–4	2	3	2	1	2
History of venous thromboembolic disease	4	4	2	2	2	1	2
Migraine with focal neurological symptoms	2–3	2–3	1–2	2	2	1	2
HIV positive	1	1	1	1	1	3	3
Non-vascular disease diabetes	2	2	2	2	2	1	2

(Continued)

TABLE 7.3 Medical eligibility criteria for selected family planning methods (World Health Organization) (Continued)

Condition	Combined oral	Combined injectable	Progestogen only oral	Depot progestogens	Sub-dermal implants	Copper IUD	Levonorgestrel IUD
Diabetes with vascular disease or of > 20 years, duration	3–4	3–4	2	3	2	1	2
History of cholestasis	2–3	2	1–2	1–2	1–2	1	1–2
Cancer of cervix	2	2	1	2	2	2–4	2–4
Cancer of breast	3–4	3–4	3–4	3–4	3–4	1	3–4
Cancer of ovary	1	1	1	1	1	2–3	2–3
PID	1	1	1	1	1	2–4	2–4

Classification categories:
1. A condition for which there is no restriction for the use of the contraceptive method.
2. A condition where the advantages of using the method generally outweigh the theoretical or proven risks.
3. A condition where the theoretic or proven risks usually outweigh the advantages of using the method.
4. A condition which represents an unacceptable health risk if the contraceptive method is used.

IUCD (FIG 7.1)

The main mechanism of action of the IUD is the reduction in the number of viable gametes, particularly sperm but also oocytes. The classification is outlined in Table 7.4.

Benefits
The IUCD is a highly effective method of contraception with virtually no systemic side-effects, and so it can be used by breast-feeding mothers.

Side-effects
There may be some dysmenorrhoea, and bleeding is increased by an average of 40% (but much reduced with the levonorgestrel IUCD, see page 268). The risk of ectopic pregnancy is reduced overall, but if pregnancy does occur it is more likely to be ectopic than if the IUCD was not present. The risk of PID is small and limited only to the first few weeks after insertion. Mild infection can be treated with the IUCD in situ, but if the device is removed because of infection it should not be re-inserted for 6 months. Asymptomatic actinomycoses on a smear test does not require treatment, but if there is any tenderness on VE, remove the IUCD and treat with high-dose penicillin for several weeks.

Contraindications
These include previous tubal pregnancy and PID. (If the patient is symptom free, and the PID was not severe, occurred > 6 months previously and has not subsequently recurred, then this may be only a relative contraindication.) The use of IUCDs is also contraindicated in pregnancy, the immunosuppressed, those with a distorted uterine cavity, Wilson's disease or a past history of bacterial endocarditis or prosthetic valve replacement. It is relatively contraindicated with HIV infection.

TABLE 7.4 Classification of IUCDs

	Coil	Lasts for
2nd generation	Multiload Cu250 Nova T (Novagard)	3–5 years
3rd generation	Multiload Cu375 Copper Cu380 (slimline)	5 + years
4th generation	GyneFix frameless IUCD Levonorgestrel System	5 years 5 years

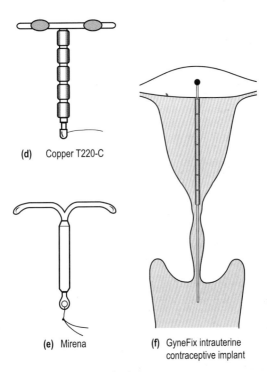

(a) Multiload 375   **(b)** Copper 7   **(c)** Nova T

(d) Copper T220-C

(e) Mirena

(f) GyneFix intrauterine contraceptive implant

Fig. 7.1 Intrauterine contraceptive devices.

Insertion

This requires training. Ideally, IUCDs should be inserted between days 1 and 7 of the cycle (earlier carries a higher expulsion rate, later and there may already be a viable pregnancy). They may also be inserted at the time of TOP (although the expulsion rate is higher) or 6 weeks postpartum. Perform a speculum and pelvic examination, looking particularly for the position of the uterus, its size and the presence of fibroids. Under speculum visualization, and ideally in lithotomy, pass a sound to determine the length of the uterus and then place the IUCD at the fundus (it may be necessary to grasp the cervix with a Vulsellum or Rampley's sponge-holding forceps). Cut the threads to 3 cm and arrange for follow-up at 1 and 6 weeks to check the threads. The technique for inserting GyneFix is different, as the knot in the string needs to be embedded in the fundus; insertion is simple but requires appropriate training.

Lost thread

Arrange an USS to confirm that the IUCD has not been expelled and that it is still inside the uterine cavity. Insert a thread retrieval hook to try and bring the threads down. If this is not successful, remove the device with artery forceps or similar; a GA is sometimes required. Hysteroscopy may be of help. If the coil is in the abdominal cavity, it should be sought and removed as it may lead to an intense inflammatory reaction. Although inert devices (e.g. SAF-T coil and Lippes Loop) are no longer available, some women may still have them in situ and they may be deeply embedded.

Pregnancy

More than 90% of pregnancies are intrauterine. The problem with leaving an IUCD in situ is the increased risk of second trimester miscarriage (up to 50%) and later problems from APH, stillbirth and preterm delivery. The coil should be removed in the first trimester, as this carries a lower overall risk. Do not attempt thread retrieval if the threads have been drawn up, but treat as a 'high-risk' pregnancy.

Removal

Start alternative methods of contraception before removal. The IUCD should be changed every 3–5 years (see Table 7.4) unless the woman is aged ≥ 40 years when the device is inserted, in which cause she can keep it until 1 year after her last menstrual period (i.e. menopause). The coil should ideally be left in situ after sterilization until after the next menstrual period.

COMBINED ORAL CONTRACEPTIVE (TABLE 7.5)

This acts mainly by inhibiting ovulation. The tablets are taken daily for 21 days followed by a 7-day break during which there is a withdrawal bleed. It should be started on the first day of the cycle, or 3 weeks postpartum, or on the same day as a termination or miscarriage.

Benefits
Oral contraceptives are very effective means of reversible contraception. They reduce blood loss and decrease the incidence of dysmenorrhoea, fibroids, ectopic pregnancy, endometriosis, functional ovarian cysts, ovarian cancer (by 40%), endometrial cancer (by 50%) and PID (due to increased mucus viscosity).

Side-effects
These are weight gain, breast tenderness, changes in libido, and an increase in the incidence of MI, stroke and venous thromboembolic disease.

- The risk of MI is not increased in pill users who do not smoke and who do not have either hypertension or diabetes, regardless of age. Hypertension increases the risk three-fold and smoking increases the risk ten-fold in COC users.
- The risk of ischaemic stroke is increased by 1.5 at all ages, but that of haemorrhagic stroke is not increased until > 35 years. Hypertension increases the risk of both (three- and ten-fold, respectively) and smoking increases the risk three-fold over that of non-users.
- The risk of venous thromboembolic disease is increased three- to six-fold in pill users over non-users and is unrelated to oestrogen if the dose is < 50 μg ethinylestradiol. Risks are unrelated to smoking or hypertension. Pills containing desogestrel and gestodene probably carry a small risk of venous thromboembolic disease above pills containing levonorgestrel. Desogestrel and gestodene were originally used because of their favourable effects on serum markers for cardiovascular and cerebrovascular disease, but there are insufficient data to show whether these benefits translate into a genuine clinical benefit. It is therefore advised that they should not be used by women with risk factors for thromboembolism including BMI > 30 kg/m^2, varicose veins, immobility or family history of thrombosis.
- The relative risk of breast cancer with COC users is 1.24, but there is a decreased risk of metastases (RR = 0.8). The relationship

TABLE 7.5 Classification of combined oral contraceptives

Ethinyl estradiol	Pill	Progestogen	Dose (mg)	Notes
20 mcgs	Mercilon	Desogestrel	0.15	Particularly suitable for the obese or older woman. Desogestrel has been reported to → better cycle control than norethisterone
	Loestrin 20	Norethisterone	1	
30 mcgs	Marvelon	Desogestrel	0.15	Desogestrel and gestodene may have less adverse effects on lipids than levonorgestrel and norethisterone. There may, however, be an increased risk of venous thromboembolism (see text)
	Femodene (± ED)	Gestodene	0.075	
	Minulet			
	Microgynon 30 (± ED)	Levonorgestrel	0.15	
	Ovranette			
	Eugynon 30	Levonorgestrel	0.25	
	Ovran 30			
	Loestrin 30	Norethisterone	1.5	
35 mcgs	Brevinor	Norethisterone	0.5	
	Ovysmen			
	Norimin	Norethisterone	1	
	Cilest	Norgestimate	0.25	Norgestimate may have less adverse effects on lipids than norethisterone, but probably similar effects on venous thromboembolic disease as gestodene
50 mcgs	Ovran	Levonorgestrel	0.25	For circumstances with reduced bio-availability, e.g. while using enzyme-inducing drugs. There is an increased possibility of side-effects
	Norinyl – 1	Norethisterone	1	

between the pill and breast cancer, therefore, remains unclear (increased detection or actual effect?).

Overall, COC use does not increase or decrease mortality – there is a lower death rate from ovarian carcinoma and a higher rate of mortality from circulatory disorders and cervical carcinoma. These effects are seen with those taking the pill and in the 10 years afterwards.

Contraindications

These include pregnancy, severe or multiple risk factors for arterial disease, a history of arterial or venous thrombosis, IIID, severe hypertension, focal migraine, severe migraine, crescendo migraine, TIA, liver disorders, breast or genital tract carcinoma, history of HUS, or during pregnancy of pemphygoid gestationis, pruritus, chorea or cholestatic jaundice. The COC should not be taken by breast-feeding mothers as it interferes with lactation. Death due to the pill in those > 35 years old is 8 times more common in those women who smoke, and either the pill or the smoking should be stopped at this age. Low-risk non-smokers may continue the COC until the menopause (although they will not know when this is without stopping it!).

Management
Check ups

The woman should be seen usually at 3 months and thereafter every 6 months to have a BP check, discuss side-effects and ensure that she is up to date with her cervical smears. The objective is to achieve good cycle control with the lowest possible dose of oestrogen.

Breakthrough bleeding This may take up to 6 months to resolve after starting a COC. It is uncertain whether this represents an increased risk of failure. Check compliance, a pregnancy test and exclude cervical pathology by speculum examination. Take a drug history (see Effectiveness, below). Then change to a pill with an increased dose of oestrogen, or return to an older Gestogen, or try a phasic pill.

Forgotten pill The pill should be taken as soon as it is remembered, and the next one again at the normal time. If the pill is taken more than 12 hours late, additional contraceptive methods are required for the next 7 days (e.g. condom). If these 7 days run past the end of the packet, the next packet should be started at once without leaving a gap. (If 'every day' [ED] pills are being used, the woman should miss out the seven inactive pills.) *The most critical time for missing pills is at the start of a packet (i.e. lengthening the pill-free interval).* If two or more pills are missed in the first 7 days, consider PCC.

Effectiveness This is reduced by liver enzyme inducers (most anticonvulsants, griseofulvin and rifampicin); therefore use a 50 µg ethinylestradiol preparation. Vomiting and use of antibiotics may interfere with absorption, and additional precautions should be used for 7 days. Diarrhoea alone is not a significant problem.

PROGESTOGEN ONLY CONTRACEPTIVES

The progestogen only pill (POP)

The pill is taken every day as close to the same time as possible (within a 3-hour window) and it acts on cervical mucus and alters the endometrium. The Gestogen dose is lower than in the COC and there is no oestrogen. Ovulation is inhibited in only ≈ 50%, and 20–25% have functional ovarian cysts (usually asymptomatic). The main side-effect is irregular bleeding, or occasionally, amenorrhoea. The overall ectopic risk is reduced, but if pregnancy does occur it is more likely to be an ectopic than if the POP was not being taken. Unlike the COC, it is not contraindicated in breast-feeding and may be used in those with diabetes, hypertension and smokers > 35 years old. Side-effects include nausea, vomiting, headache, breast discomfort, depression, skin disorders and weight changes. There is no significant increase in the risk of venous thromboembolic disease. For the different types of pill available, see Table 7.6.

If a pill is missed (i.e. it is outside the 3-hour window) it should be taken as soon as it is remembered, and the next one taken at its usual time. If the pill was more than 3 hours overdue, additional protection should be used for the next 7 days. Vomiting may interfere with absorption, so that additional precautions should again be used for 7 days.

EMERGENCY CONTRACEPTION

Levonorgestrel alone (0.75 mg twice, separated by 12 hours) is more effective and has fewer side-effects than the Yuzpe method (two tablets, each with ethinylestradiol 50 µg and levonorgestrel 250 µg repeated again 12 hours later). If tablets are vomited, an extra two should be taken. The pills inhibit or delay ovulation, can be used up to 72 hours after intercourse and prevent 75% of pregnancies which would have occurred that cycle. The next 'period' may be early, on time or late, and barrier contraception should be used until then. If there has been no 'period' after 3–4 weeks, a pregnancy test must be arranged (pregnancy after postcoital contraception is not in itself an indication for TOP as there have been no reported teratogenic problems).

TABLE 7.6 Classification of progestogen-only contraceptives		
Progestogen	*Pill*	*Dose (mg)*
Norethisterone type	Micronor	0.35
	Noriday	0.35
	Femulen	0.5
Levonorgestrel type	Microval	0.03
	Norgeston	0.03
	Neogest	0.075

An IUCD can be inserted up to 5 days after the estimated day of ovulation (which may be > 5 days after intercourse) and has an almost 100% success rate in preventing pregnancy that cycle.

Mifepristone, in a dose of 600 mg or less, is also effective in emergency contraception but is not licensed.

INJECTABLE PROGESTOGENS

These carry a failure rate of 0–1 : 100 woman-years. Depo Provera (150 mg medroxyprogesterone acetate IM 12 weekly) is commonly used. About 80% of women will be amenorrhoeic by 1 year, although 2% will develop troublesome menorrhagia. As heavy bleeding can occur, Depo Provera is best left until 6 weeks postpartum, using other methods from 3 to 6 weeks. Delayed return to fertility may occur, lasting up to 18 months. Most women gain some weight. Recent studies suggest that the effect on reduced bone mineral density is unlikely to be clinically significant, but concerns remain about its use in adolescents who have yet to reach their peak bone mass. It should also perhaps be discontinued in those > 45 years old for the same reason.

IMPLANTS

Implanon is a single rod (around the size of a matchstick), with a disposable inserter, containing desogestrel at a dose that inhibits ovulation. Irregular bleeding occurs relatively commonly. It lasts 3 years and has a very low failure rate.

BARRIER METHODS

These reduce the transmission of most STIs with both vaginal and anal intercourse.

Condoms These are effective when used properly and with spermicidal cream. The risk of bursting is reduced if air is expelled from the teat. Manufacturers are now producing different sizes, which may help with recurrent bursting.

Diaphragms These stretch from the posterior fornix to above the symphysis pubis (like ring pessaries) whereas cervical caps fit over the cervix (which needs to be prominent). They should be used with spermicide, inserted < 2 hours before intercourse and removed at least 6 hours later. Side-effects include UTIs and problems with rubber hypersensitivity.

Female condoms These condoms (e.g. Femidom) have a high failure rate, usually due to the penis being inserted between the condom and the vaginal wall.

STERILIZATION

Consider which partner should be sterilized. How stable is the relationship? If the woman is obese, it may be technically difficult to undertake laparoscopy. Legally, consent is only required from the person wishing to be sterilized. Preoperative counselling details are outlined below and these details must be recorded in the notes:

- Irreversibility and alternative methods of contraception (10% regret their decision at 18 months and 1% seek reversal, especially those who are single and younger).
- Failure rates and, in women, the risk of ectopic pregnancy.
- A woman should be aware that if laparoscopy is unsuccessful or if there are complications, it might be necessary to perform a laparotomy under the same GA.
- After sterilization in men, it is necessary to wait until two clear semen specimens have been obtained (months) before other contraception is stopped. In women, it is necessary to continue with alternative contraception until the next menstrual period.

Female sterilization

This is usually carried out laparoscopically by tubal occlusion (Falope rings, Hulka clips, Filshie clips or diathermy) but can be performed by laparotomy, at caesarean section or, more radically, by hysterectomy. Tubal occlusion after the age of 30 is not associated with an increase in abdominal pain, dyspareunia or menstrual disturbance; there is debate about this possibility before this age, although it is possible that menstrual disturbance has been masked by the COC prior to the operation.

Male sterilization

Vasectomy can be performed on an outpatient basis under local anaesthesia. Bruising and haematoma formation are not uncommon. The failure rate is 1 : 1000 following two negative semen samples. The evidence suggests that the incidence of testicular cancer is not increased, although there is still some concern about the risk of prostate cancer.

DEVELOPMENTAL PROBLEMS

DELAYED PUBERTY AND PRIMARY AMENORRHOEA

In normal development there is a trigger which leads to the pulsatile release of LH and FSH between the ages of 5 and 10 years, with an ovarian response occurring usually after the age of 8 years. The first sign of puberty in girls is increased growth and, almost simultaneously, breast budding followed by the appearance of pubic hair. Menarche usually follows within 2 years of the first breast and hair development, always after, and usually within, 1 year of the peak growth velocity. Although deviation from this sequence (loss of consonance) is 'abnormal', it may occur in up to 50% of girls. Primary amenorrhoea is defined as no menstruation by the age of 14 years accompanied by failure to develop secondary sexual characteristics. It is also defined as no menstruation by the age of 16 years with normal sexual development. A paediatric endocrinology clinic is usually more appropriate for delayed puberty consultations that a gynaecology clinic.

Initial management

- Exclude pregnancy.
- Ask about chronic illnesses, anorexia, excessive fitness training or a family history of delayed puberty. Also ask about heart problems (associated with chromosomal disorders), urinary or bowel problems (associated with anatomical abnormalities of the genital tract), hernia repairs (gonadal disorder) and general development (slow in hypothyroidism).
- Carry out an examination, especially height and weight, the presence of secondary sexual characteristics, hirsutism, virilization and visual fields (a vaginal examination should only be considered

in sexually active girls). Look for signs of dysharmonious development (e.g. pubic hair but no breast development) and for signs of Turner's syndrome.

- Serum for LH and FSH (low with constitutional delay), testosterone (increased in polycystic ovarian syndrome), free T_4, TSH (increased in primary hypothyroidism) and Prl (the patient should ideally be unstressed for Prl levels).
- Consider a karyotype.
- Consider obtaining an X-ray for bone age if constitutional delay is suspected.

Causes and further management

Normal secondary sexual characteristics but primary amenorrhoea

This is most commonly caused by an imperforate hymen and is characterized by cyclical pain and a haematocolpos. A cruciate incision, usually under anaesthesia, is all that is required. Much more rarely, there is a horizontal septae or an absent uterus (see p. 230). A progesterone challenge test will identify constitutional menstrual delay (i.e. will result in bleeding only if the oestradiol level and genital tract is normal). Give Provera 10 mg TID PO for 10 days, or Gestone 100–200 mg IM stat. There should be a withdrawal bleed within 10–14 days of the injection or 10–14 days after stopping the oral progestogen.

Poor or absent secondary sexual characteristics

Constitutional delay The diagnosis is likely in a healthy adolescent who is short for the family but appropriate for the stage of puberty and bone age. There is often a family history and it may be associated with chronic systemic disease (rare, but consider decreased T_4 and malabsorption). If the X-ray bone age is less than the chronological age then it is reasonable to adopt a conservative approach. Anorexia nervosa should also be considered.

Ovarian dysfunction This may be due to gonadal agenesis with Turner's syndrome (see p. 9) or Turner's mosaic. Treatment is specialized, as oestrogen treatment may predispose to short stature by premature epiphyseal closure. Therapy is with ethinylestradiol, initially 1–2 µg/day PO increasing to 10 µg/day over the next 18 months. A progestogen (e.g. norethisterone 350 µg/day) is then added for 5 days every 4 weeks. The dose of oestrogen is increased to 20–30 µg/day and COC substituted. The polycystic ovarian syndrome (see p. 244) may occasionally present as primary amenorrhoea.

Hypothalamopituitary disorders Hypogonadotrophic hypogonadism is usually associated with pituitary tumours and other pituitary deficiencies. In Kallmann syndrome there is a congenital deficiency of LHRH and absent olfactory sensation. Hypothyroidism is likely to cause pubertal delay. Hyperprolactinaemia is rare.

INTERSEX DISORDERS AND AMBIGUOUS GENITALIA

Early multidisciplinary subspecialist involvement is essential, particularly surrounding the issues of genital surgery and gender assignment. There will be initial shock at the diagnosis, with possible subsequent depression, doubts of gender, concerns over fertility, issues of sexuality, cultural problems and a sense of worthlessness. Peer support from those with similar problems is important.

In those with XY chromosomes, testosterone masculinizes the otherwise female external genitalia and stimulates the mesonephric (Wolffian) system to develop. Mullerian inhibitory factor inhibits the paramesonephric (Mullerian) system, which would otherwise form female internal genitalia.

XY but look female (male pseudohermaphroditism)

Testicular feminization syndrome (androgen insensitivity) This is an XL recessive disorder due to the absence of androgen receptors. There are complete and incomplete forms. Presentation is usually after puberty, with amenorrhoea in the presence of normal breast development, scanty pubic and axillary hair, a blind-ending vagina, absent uterus, and female habitus and psychosexual orientation. Gonadectomy is essential because of the risk of malignant change; this should probably be done before puberty and followed by an exogenous hormone puberty induction.

5α-reductase deficiency. There is an AR target enzyme defect. At puberty, considerable, but still incomplete, virilization occurs, with male body habitus, psychosexual orientation and gender conversion.

Failure of testicular development This may occur with true gonadal agenesis. The internal and external genitalia are female. This is rare.

PRE-PUBERTAL PROBLEMS

See also Primary amenorrhoea (p. 227) and Ambiguous genitalia (p. 229).

Vaginal discharge

Such a symptom raises the possibility of, but does not necessarily imply, sexual abuse.

- Non-microbial causes. Threadworms are possible. Foreign-body insertion is rare.
- Microbial causes. Investigation is difficult to interpret as there are little data on the commensal profile of children. In those with discharge, the GpA streptococcus is commonly found, followed by *H. influenzae* and candida. Bowel flora are also common. Gardnerella and *Trichomonas vaginalis* are probably not commensals. Swabs should also be checked for chlamydia and *Neisseria gonorrhoea*.

SEXUAL ABUSE

> ⚠ There are numerous pitfalls to the clinical examination, and you may be expected to demonstrate a depth of experience in court which you do not actually have. Early senior multidisciplinary help is essential in this highly emotive area where incorrect interpretation of the signs can have major consequences. A colposcope is important and photographic records are essential.

Sexual abuse is the involvement of dependent sexually immature children and adolescents in sexual activity they do not truly comprehend and to which they are unable to give informed consent and which violates social taboos or family roles. The abuser is usually male and well known to the child and family. It may present acutely, following injury or allegation, or may be suggested by precociousness, self-harming (usually in older children/teenagers, and may include drugs and prostitution), eating disorders, enuresis, encopresis, sleep problems, lowered achievements, psychosomatic problems and attention-seeking behaviour.

The history should be carefully taken and documented, and the social work team involved if appropriate. Examination, which usually does not require anaesthetic, should involve specialists and may include paediatricians and a police surgeon, particularly in the acute situation. Swabs (which may include swabs for DNA analysis) should be taken with a 'secure chain of evidence' in case this is required for a later legal action. Look for bleeding, bruising or any other area of injury, particularly lacerations at the posterior fourchette and perineal abrasions. A normal hymen has a number of different shapes (annular, crescentic, fimbriated, septate, sleeve or funnel shaped). Notches and clefts can be highly suggestive of penetrating injury, but may be normal if associated with an intravaginal ridge above them; they are very rare in the posterior segment in non-abused girls. Straddle injuries very rarely affect the hymen, and there is much more likely to be bruising anterior to the vagina or laterally (e.g. labia majora). It is also rare for tampon use to cause hymenal injury (although it may increase the diameter slightly), and there are no reported cases of congenital absence of the hymen. A normal prepubertal hymen does not exclude abuse.

ECTOPIC PREGNANCY

> This refers to any non-intrauterine pregnancy and, although the pregnancies may be ovarian, cervical or intra-abdominal, the vast majority are tubal. The incidence of tubal pregnancy is 1 : 200–400 pregnancies, with 50% occurring in the ampulla, 28% in the isthmus and rest either fimbrial or interstitial. There may be a history of a previous ectopic pregnancy, previous surgery, PID, endometriosis or IVF, but more than 50% occur in those with no predisposing risk factors.

Clinical features

Clinical features range from no symptoms at all, to right, left or bilateral lower abdominal pain, PV bleeding, intra-abdominal haemorrhage (peritonism and shoulder tip pain) and collapse. Pelvic examinations should be gentle to avoid tubal rupture. A positive pregnancy test in the absence of a demonstrable intrauterine pregnancy should always be considered to be an ectopic pregnancy until proven otherwise. Intra-abdominal pregnancies are exceedingly rare, but have progressed to term to be delivered by laparotomy (do not attempt to remove the placenta).

Investigations

An USS is most useful in demonstrating an intrauterine pregnancy. A gestational sac may be confused with a pseudosac (due to thickened endometrium), which is seen in 20% of ectopic pregnancies and which lacks the echogenic ring of a gestational sac (see Figs 7.2–7.4). A true

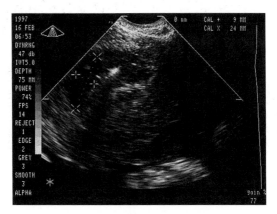

Fig. 7.2 Pseudosac with IUCD in situ. Ectopic pregnancy at laparoscopy.

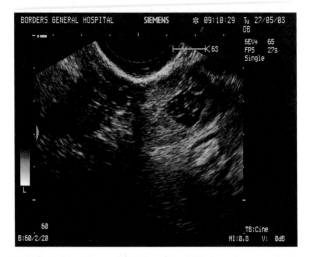

Fig. 7.3 An ectopic pregnancy with cardiac activity.

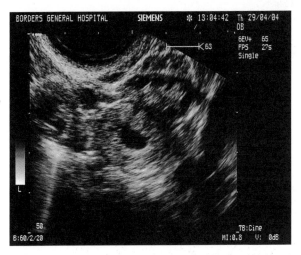

Fig. 7.4 A thickened fallopian tube containing blood from an ectopic pregnancy (the 'doughnut' sign).

sac is usually smooth, eccentrically placed, has a double rim and may contain a yolk sac. It may be possible to see an adnexal gestational sac (which may or may not contain a yolk sac, fetal pole or FH), blood clot in the tube or blood in the pouch of Douglas. The absence of adnexal findings on USS, however, does not exclude an ectopic pregnancy. Check a chlamydia swab.

Management

Management depends on the overall clinical picture, the scan result and the serum hCG:

- If the patient is collapsed, shocked and has a positive pregnancy test, set up two IV infusions and crossmatch 6 units of RCC. Infuse colloid, crystalloid and, afterwards, if necessary, O negative or un-crossmatched group-specific blood. Arrange theatre urgently.
- If there is a positive pregnancy test with clinical signs of an ectopic pregnancy (pelvic tenderness, cervical excitation, shoulder tip pain) and an empty uterus on TV ultrasound, carry out a diagnostic laparoscopy.
- If there is a positive pregnancy test, an empty uterus and no clinical signs, check a quantitative hCG. If > 1000 IU following a TV scan or > 6500 IU following a TA scan, consider laparoscopy.

Otherwise, repeat after at least 48 hours, as above. If less than doubling, or steady, or only slightly reduced, consider laparoscopy to exclude ectopic pregnancy.

● If the hCG levels are falling rapidly, the pregnancy (whether an intrauterine or ectopic) is aborting. If the patient is well, conservative management is often appropriate, with further hCG checks to ensure that the level continues to fall.

Laparoscopy may be warranted if symptoms develop.

Treatment

Surgical treatment may be carried out laparoscopically or at laparotomy. Laparotomy is preferred if there is significant haemodynamic compromise. Laparoscopy has the advantage of a shorter hospital stay and quicker recovery time over laparotomy; subsequent reproductive outcome is similar.

The surgery can be either by salpingectomy (removal of the tube) or salpingostomy (a linear incision is made over the ectopic using unipolar needlepoint diathermy, the ectopic removed, and the tube left to close spontaneously). Salpingectomy is preferable to salpingotomy when the contralateral tube is healthy as it is associated with a lower rate of persisting trophoblast and subsequent repeat ectopic while having a similar intrauterine pregnancy rate (*www.cochrane.co.uk* 2004). Salpingotomy is reasonable when there is only one tube but is associated with a 20% rate of further ectopic. Salpingectomy is indicated in the presence of uncontrollable bleeding, recurrent ectopic in the same tube, or when childbearing is complete. With a fimbrial ectopic it might also be possible to 'milk' the pregnancy from the tube at laparotomy, or tease it out through the fimbrial end laparoscopically.

If the tube is conserved it is essential to ensure that the hCG is falling; if not, there is likely to be residual trophoblast. The hCG should fall to 25% of the pretreatment level within 4 days of surgery (average time to an undetectable level is 4 weeks).

Medical management of ectopic pregnancy is also an option. One method is to give methotrexate (e.g. at a dose of 50 mg/m² IM) without folate rescue, providing the patient is haemodynamically stable, any USS visualized ectopic is < 3.5 cm and there are no blood or liver problems (see protocol in Amer J Obstet Gynecol 1993;168:1759).

As the risk of recurrence of further ectopic pregnancies is around 10%, it is important that advice be given to present early (around 5–6 weeks) in all future pregnancies to ensure that the pregnancy is intrauterine.

ENDOMETRIOSIS

Endometriosis is present in 10–25% of women presenting with gynaecological symptoms. The commonest sites are the ovary (55%), posterior broad ligament (35%), anterior and posterior pouch of Douglas (34%) and uterosacral ligaments (28%). There is a great variation in symptoms, and there is poor correlation between symptoms and laparoscopic findings. Pain is usually associated with menstruation or may occur immediately premenstrually. Dyspareunia is common. There may rarely be rupture or torsion of an endometrioma, irregular menses or, rarely, cyclical problems with rectal bleeding, tenesmus, diarrhoea, constipation, haemoptysis, dysuria, ureteric colic or scar pains.

The chance of successful pregnancy may be as low as half that of the normal population. This may be due to an endocrinopathy, reduced frequency of coitus, tubal dysfunction, early pregnancy failure or reduced sperm function (secretions are luteolytic and the increased numbers of macrophages are highly phagocytic to sperm). Laparoscopically, endometriosis may appear white or red (active lesions), as black/brown 'powder' burns or as white plaques of old collagen. There may also be circular defects in the peritoneum or endometriomas, with 'chocolate' fluid containing debris from cyclical menstruation.

Medical treatment principles
Drug treatment is not indicated for the treatment of asymptomatic, minimal or minor endometriosis in patients wishing to conceive. For symptomatic relief in such patients, treatment should be limited to 3 months. Other symptomatic treatment includes analgesia, tranexamic acid and the Mirena IUCD. If direct treatment is required, there are two therapeutic options: pseudopregnancy and pseudomenopause. Recurrence after such treatments is common. Contraception is advisable (e.g. with barrier methods) unless using the COC. To avoid inadvertent administration during pregnancy, all therapies should be initiated within the first 3 days of the start of a menstrual period.

Pseudo-pregnancy For symptomatic endometriosis, continuous progestogen therapy, e.g. medroxyprogesterone acetate (Provera) 10 mg TID for 90 days, is most cost-effective, has fewer side-effects

> 10 mm. Serum levels correlate well with tumour size, a macroadenoma usually secreting at least 2500–3000 mU/l. If the Prl level is < 2000–3000 mU/l with a tumour > 10 mm, then pituitary stalk compression from a non-secreting macroadenoma or other tumour is possible (e.g. a craniopharyngioma). If the Prl level is > 8000 mU/l, an adenoma is likely. If there is a macroadenoma, also check visual fields and arrange a short Synacthen test. One-third of adenomas regress spontaneously and < 5% of microadenomas become macroadenomas.

Secondary hyperprolactinaemia
Outside pregnancy and lactation, this may occur secondary to primary hypothyroidism, chronic renal failure, stalk compression, PCOS or drugs (phenothiazines, haloperidol, metoclopramide, cimetidine, methyldopa, antihistamines, morphine). The modern lower doses of oestrogen in the COC do not usually elevate prolactin. Around 10% of those with PCOS also have an elevated prolactin level, although the mechanism remains obscure.

Idiopathic hyperprolactinaemia
This may be due to microadenomas not picked up by MRI. Prl levels are usually < 2500 mU/l. The condition should still be treated as there is a risk of reduced libido and (if there is amenorrhoea) osteoporosis. HRT should only be considered in those with treated microadenomas and given only under very close supervision.

Treatment of adenomas or idiopathic hyperprolactinaemia
Medical treatment is with dopamine agonists. Cabergoline 0.25 mg twice weekly (increasing to a maximum of 1 mg twice weekly) is more effective and has fewer side-effects than bromocriptine (nausea, vomiting, postural hypotension). The Prl level returns to normal (aim for 200–300 mU/L) in 90% of patients, with restoration of periods in 70%. Treatment reduces the tumour size (and induces fibrosis), although the size often increases again after treatment is stopped. Although there are no recognized teratogenic problems with either preparation, there are only limited data on pregnancy safety and they should be stopped. Surgical treatment with transnasal transsphenoidal microsurgical excision is rarely used and is reserved for those tumours resistant to medical therapy.

Pregnancy and lactation
In pregnancy, discontinue dopamine agonist treatment as soon as pregnancy is confirmed. The high levels of pregnancy-related prolactin

render prolactin measurement of little value as a disease marker. There is a risk of tumour expansion in pregnancy, probably < 5% with macroadenomas and < 2% with microadenomas. In those known previously to have macroadenomas, arrange regular formal visual field testing. Those with microadenomas should probably simply be reviewed and advised to attend if there are headaches or visual-field symptoms. Breast-feeding is not contraindicated.

INFECTIONS

PELVIC INFLAMMATORY DISEASE (PID)

> The UK incidence is 1–2% per year amongst sexually active women, although this decreases with increasing age. It is associated with early age at first intercourse, and is less likely with COC and condom use. Infection ascends, possibly assisted by proteolytic enzymes and the motility of sperm or protozoa, to cause a primary infection. This may recur (either through reactivation or by repeated exposure) or may become chronic following secondary infection with endogenous organisms (usually polymicrobial). Infection may progress to pelvic abscess formation. Uterine instrumentation, especially at the time of TOP, also increases the risk of PID. The 'classic' picture of febrile illness, raised ESR and palpable adnexal swelling is seen in only 16% of those with laparoscopically proven PID.

If the diagnosis is based on:

- All three of
  - — abdominal tenderness
  - — cervical excitation
  - — adnexal tenderness
- and at least one of
  - — T > 38°C
  - — WCC > 10×10^9/l
  - — ESR > 15 mm/h

then 70% will have salpingitis, 30% adhesions and 6% tubal occlusion at laparoscopy. Between 40% and 50% will be chlamydia positive.

There may also be:

- irregular PV bleeding (in 33%)
- vaginal discharge (in 50%)
- elevated CRP (80%).

The true incidence of PID is likely to be higher than cases identified using these criteria as a significant proportion of cases, particularly those with chlamydia, may have minimal symptoms or signs. Peak prevalence is at 15–25 years of age, raising important questions about whether this age group should be screened for subclinical chlamydial infection (ideally using first-pass urine samples for PCR/LCR). Those undergoing induced abortion should be either screened for infection and treated before the procedure, or receive prophylactic antibiotics. It is also probable that those undergoing uterine instrumentation (including IUCD insertion, infertility laparoscopy and endometrial sampling), particularly in the 15–25 year age group, would benefit from screening.

Investigations
Take a history, carry out a clinical examination and check the WCC, ESR ± CRP. An endocervical swab (rotated to ensure that cells are taken) should be checked for chlamydia (or first-pass urine for LCR/PCR if available) and a further endocervical swab placed in Amies transport medium prior to culture for both *Neisseria gonorrhoeae* and anaerobes. Although the gold standard test for PID is laparoscopic evidence of tubal inflammation, laparoscopy is usually only carried out if there is a pelvic mass, failure to respond to treatment, or significant doubt about the diagnosis.

Laparoscopic findings are as follows:

- Mild: hyperaemia, exudate, oedema with freely mobile tubes.
- Moderate: gross exudate with adherent tubes.
- Severe: tubo-ovarian mass, pyosalpinx or abscess.

Although many primary and most secondary infections are polymicrobial, some infections may fit specific syndromes (Table 7.10).

Treatment
Initial treatment is usually blind, as delay in treatment increases the risks of infertility. (See p. 253 for specific treatment after identification of the organism.)

The choice of oral or IV treatment depends on the patient's condition:

TABLE 7.10 Infections associated with PID

Organism	Age of patient	Length of illness	Temp.	Features
Chlamydia trachomatis	Young	7 days to several months	Usually normal	Often minimal clinical features but there may be intermenstrual bleeding or urinary symptoms. Dyspareunia is also common
Anaerobes	Older	< 3 days	> 38°C	Often 2nd or 3rd infection. Often unwell
Neisseria gonorrhoea	Young	< 3 days	> 38°C	Is rare in the UK Unwell and very tender
Streptococci, coagulase negative staphylococci and actinomycoses				Are rare

- If the patient is clinically well:
  — doxycycline 100 mg BD PO for 14–28 days (or azithromycin 1 g stat. PO, see p. 254), plus
  — metronidazole 200 mg TID PO for 14–28 days.
- If the patient is clinically unwell:
  — azithromycin 1 g stat. PO (or doxycycline 100 mg BD PO for 14–28 days), plus
  — either cefuroxime 750 mg IV TID (or gentamicin IV, see p. 129) and metronidazole 500 mg IV TID or co-amoxiclav 1.2 g IV TID.

Long-term prognosis
There is a seven- to tenfold increase in the risk of ectopic pregnancy. The incidence of tubal infertility increases with increasing numbers of infections and is > 50% in those who have had three or more infections. Contact tracing of chlamydia-positive patients is important as treatment of partners reduces the risk of new and recurrent cases. Treatment of asymptomatic chlamydia-positive women also reduces the incidence of PID. One-third of patients will have a recurrence within 1 year.

VAGINAL DISCHARGE

> **Physiological vaginal discharge changes throughout the reproductive life, increasing as the oestrogen level increases (e.g. at puberty, in pregnancy or with the COC).**

History
Is the discharge itchy (candida) or offensive (foreign body, *Trichomonas vaginalis* or bacterial vaginosis)? Is there any pain or fever (PID if abdominal pain, HSV if vulval pain)? A sexual history should be obtained, and if there is a new sexual partner the possibility of a STI arises. If so, consider referral to a genitourinary medicine clinic for diagnosis, treatment and contact tracing.

Management
Perform a speculum examination to see whether the discharge is vaginal or cervical:

- If the history is one of pruritus vulvae, the patient is well and the discharge is white, prescribe antifungal preparations (swabs for culture are optional). Treatment is with clotrimazole (e.g. Canesten) pessaries 200 mg nocte for 3 nights or a single 500 mg pessary stat. ± clotrimazole cream applied BD. Fluconazole (Diflucan) 150 mg/day PO stat. is also effective, but may have systemic side-effects, and should not be used in pregnancy (see Candida infection, p. 254).
- If there is a creamy yellow discharge with an offensive smell, treat with metronidazole 200 mg TID PO for 7 days or with 2% clindamycin cream 5 g applicator nocte PV for 7 nights (see Bacterial vaginosis below and *Trichomonas vaginalis*, p. 256).
- If there is no response to the above, or there are concerns about STIs, or there is an endocervical discharge, take swabs:
  — endocervical (Amies transport medium) for *N. gonorrhoea*
  — high vaginal (Amies transport medium) for routine culture
  — endocervical for *Chlamydia trachomatis* (or first-pass urine for PCR/LCR if available) and treat individual infections as outlined below
  — if you have the experience, examination of a fresh wet smear may demonstrate *T. vaginalis*.
- If there has been no response to the above measures and there are no identifiable organisms, it is worth formally calling a halt to

investigations and reviewing the original history. Discussion about the changing nature of a physiological discharge and reassurance about the absence of infection is often reassuring.

Treating a cervical ectropion to cure vaginal discharge is frequently unrewarding. Topical or systemic oestrogen treatment for recurrent vaginal infections may be of help in atrophic vaginitis (e.g. postmenopausally, those on depot progestogens).

SPECIFIC PELVIC INFECTIONS AND SEXUALLY TRANSMITTED DISEASES

With the possible exception of PID, this is best managed in an STI clinic with facilities for counselling, contact tracing and on-site Gram stain and microscopy.

Actinomycoses

This is a Gram-negative bacterium which only rarely causes salpingitis, chronic tubo-ovarian abscesses and fistulae. It may occur secondary to appendicitis or with IUCD use. It is not sexually transmitted. Treat with high-dose oral or parenteral penicillin.

Bacterial vaginosis

This occurs when lactobacilli are replaced by anaerobes, particularly bacteroides species. *Gardnerella vaginalis* probably has a small role. Bacterial vaginosis is not sexually transmitted and many women are asymptomatic. The pH increases to < 4.9 making the diagnosis unlikely, and bacterial metabolites produce volatile amines with a 'fishy' odour. The discharge is green or grey, thin and offensive. On wet microscopy there are epithelial cells surrounded by bacteria ('clue' cells). Treat with metronidazole 2 g stat. PO (or 200 mg BD for 7 days if recurrent), or with clindamycin cream 2% (5 g applicator nocte for 7 nights). If pregnant, ampicillin 500 mg PO QID may be a more appropriate oral treatment. There is no benefit in treating the partner or in using condoms.

Bacteroides spp.

These are commensals but may cause a vaginal discharge (see Bacterial vaginosis, above) or complicate pre-existing PID (leading to chronic infection). They are not sexually transmitted. Treat with metronidazole 200 mg TID 7 days or with clindamycin cream 2% (5 g applicator nocte for 7 nights).

Candida or thrush (*Candida albicans*)

This is not sexually transmitted. It presents with a whitish discharge and pruritus. The vulva and vagina may be fissured and painful. It occurs more commonly in the sexually active, the pregnant and the immunocompromised. The COC probably makes no difference. Microscopy reveals yeasts and pseudohyphae and a high vaginal swab may be cultured on Sabouraud's medium. Treatment is with clotrimazole (e.g. Canesten) pessaries 200 mg nocte for 3 nights or a single 500 mg pessary stat. ± clotrimazole cream applied BD. Fluconazole (Diflucan) 150 mg/day PO stat. is also effective, but may have systemic side-effects, and should not be used in pregnancy.

If proven infection is recurrent there is no benefit from treating the partner. Prophylactic treatment, however, may be of benefit. (For example, if the patient's symptoms are particularly troublesome premenstrually, insert a single pessary midcycle.) Alternatively, a weekly pessary may be used; 100, 200 or 500 mg, depending on which dose controls the symptoms. Natural yoghurt on a tampon nocte for 3 nights, acetic acid jelly (e.g. Aci-Jel), wiping the anus front to back, and cotton underwear may also be of help.

Chlamydia (*Chlamydia trachomatis* serovars D–K)

This is the commonest bacterial sexually transmitted infection in the UK (0.5–15% depending on sample selected), and is a much commoner cause of infection than the gonococcus. In the female it is often asymptomatic, but may cause PID, bartholinitis, spontaneous miscarriage, premature labour, neonatal conjunctivitis (5–14 days postnatally) and neonatal pneumonia. PID with associated perihepatitis is known as the Fitz–Hugh–Curtis syndrome. Reiter syndrome (arthritis, mucosal ulceration, conjunctival symptoms) is very rare in women. In the male *C. trachomatis* infection may cause urethral discharge, dysuria, epididymo-orchitis and Reiter syndrome. Diagnosis in the female is by endocervical swabs, urethral swabs or first-void urine sent in a specific transport medium for LCR or PCR.

Uncomplicated infection my be treated with azithromycin (Zithromax) 1 g (four 250 mg capsules) stat. PO (great compliance benefit), or doxycycline 200 mg stat. PO then 100 mg/day for 7 days, or erythromycin 500 mg BD for 7 days (all equally effective assuming there are no compliance problems). There is no evidence that azithromycin is adequate for chlamydial salpingitis, but it is likely that it provides adequate cover. Increased doses plus the addition of metronidazole are employed for complicated infection (see PID, p. 249). Test of cure is not essential (swabs may remain positive for up to 4 weeks despite adequate treatment), but contact tracing is important and individuals should avoid unprotected intercourse for 2 weeks.

Genital warts

These are usually caused by HPV 6 and 11, though occasionally 16 and 18. Most patients with genital HPV have no visible warts but the virus can be transmitted to sexual partners who may then develop visible lesions. Of those with warts, 25% have other demonstrable STIs. Podophyllin paint can be applied weekly to the non-pregnant patient by medical staff, with advice to wash the solution off 6 hours later. Self-treatment is also available with podophyllotoxin solution (e.g. Condyline or Warticon). This is applied BD for 3 days, repeating on a weekly cycle for 4 weeks. For patients with multiple, large warts only a few should be treated at a time, as severe discomfort has been reported. Warts may be treated with cryotherapy using liquid nitrogen, or be lasered or diathermized under GA. Immune stimulators (e.g. Imiquimod, 3M Healthcare) are occasionally considered for recalcitrant warts; treatment is expensive and not of definite proven value. Annual cervical screening is not required, but those with visible cervical warts or abnormal cytology should be colposcoped.

Gonorrhoea (*Neisseria gonorrhoea*)

The incubation period is 2–5 days for men. The vast majority of women are asymptomatic, but infection may cause PID (often at time of menstruation), urethritis, polyarthralgia, miscarriage, premature labour and neonatal ophthalmia (2–7 days postnatally). Most men have symptoms of urethritis and discharge. Swabs should be taken from the urethra and cervix and placed in Amies transport medium. A Gram stain of an endocervical swab shows Gram-negative intracellular diplococci in only 50%, so that definitive diagnosis is by culture on NYC medium. Treatment is with ampicillin 2–4 g PO stat. together with probenecid 1 g PO stat. Ciprofloxacin (Ciproxin) 250 mg PO stat. is used in penicillin allergy and for infections acquired in regions where resistance is common (take advice from the microbiology department).

Herpes (herpes simplex virus)

This infection classically occurs secondary to the sexually transmitted type II virus, but infection with type I from cold sores is increasingly common. The incubation is 2–14 days, with itch and dysuria being prominent early symptoms. The vulva becomes ulcerated and exquisitely painful and, in the first attack (which may last 3–4 weeks), there may be systemic flu-like symptoms ± secondary bacterial infection. Autoinnoculation to fingers and eyes can occur and there may be a sacral radiculopathy giving a self-limiting paraesthesia to the buttocks and thighs. Only very rarely is there an associated meningitis or encephalitis. Strong oral or IM analgesia and advice to micturate while in the bath may be of help (lidocaine [lignocaine] gel is painful to apply and may lead to hypersensitivity reactions). Aciclovir 200 mg PO 5-hourly shortens the duration of symptoms and lessens infectivity (famciclovir and valiciclovir are alternatives). Recurrent infections are shorter (lasting 5–10 days) and usually less severe. Recurrence of infection in the first year is 95% in type II and 5% in type I infections. Aciclovir cream should be used at the start of subsequent infections. Prophylactic oral aciclovir 400 mg PO BD should be reserved for those with frequent incapacitating infections (e.g. > 10/year) and should be continued for at least 12 months. There is no necessity for annual cervical cytology. (See Infection [in pregnancy], p. 186).

HIV infection
See page 195.

Lymphogranuloma venereum (tropical; *Chlamydia trachomatis* serovars L1–L3)
This is a chronic disease beginning with primary ulceration, followed 4 days to 4 months later by secondary lymphoedema and regional lymphadenitis. Treat with doxycycline 100 mg/day PO for 14 days.

Streptococci or coagulase-negative staphylococci
These may complicate pre-existing PID. Treat with ampicillin 500 mg PO QID for 7 days and metronidazole 400 mg TID for 7 days. (See Infection [in pregnancy], p. 196).

Syphilis (*Treponema pallidum*)
A primary chancre (raised, round, indurated usually painless ulcer) resolves in 3–8 weeks and may be followed by secondary fever, headaches, bone and joint pain, generalized rash, condylomata lata and generalized painless lymphadenopathy. Following the latent phase there may be tertiary gummas or quaternary neurological and cardiovascular disease. Congenital syphilis may lead to IUD or midtrimester loss. Survivors may be premature, have IUGR, Hutchinson's triad and nasal discharge. The diagnosis is made serologically, with most laboratories using the VDRL, TPHA and FTA tests. Many laboratories now screen with an antitreponemal IgG ELISA which is highly sensitive but does give false-positive results. True positive results are confirmed by the more traditional tests. Treatment is with procaine penicillin 900 mg/day IM for 10–21 days depending on the stage of the disease.

Trichomonas vaginalis
This is usually sexually transmitted. There is a foul-smelling, purulent vaginal discharge with accompanying symptoms of dysuria and vulval soreness. Diagnosis is by identification on a wet film. Treat with metronidazole as for bacterial vaginosis.

INFERTILITY

> Subfertility is an involuntary failure to conceive within
> 12 months of commencing unprotected intercourse, and may
> be primary or secondary. The incidence of primary infertility
> is at least 12% of couples. A coital history is essential. Both
> partners must be investigated.

CAUSES

The causes of infertility are given in Table 7.11. Note that the sum of
the causes in the table is > 100% as there may be more than one
factor. Many couples have subfertility with specific partners. When
there is a mild defect in one there is an increased likelihood of finding
a mild defect in the other as well.

INVESTIGATION

Female factor infertility
History
As well as a general medical, surgical and family history, take a
menstrual history and ask about galactorrhoea and hirsutism. Confirm
that the woman is taking folic acid 0.4 mg/day to reduce the incidence
of neural tube defects. Both men and women should give up smoking.
Women should not drink more than 2–4 units of alcohol per week, and
men should limit their drinking.

Examination
Check the BMI (aim for weight loss if > 30). Carry out a general
medical examination, and consider carrying out a pelvic examination
and cervical smear if appropriate.

TABLE 7.11 Causes of infertility

Female cause	Unknown cause	Male cause
15% Tubal problem	25% Idiopathic	40%
20% Anovulation	5% Sexual problem	
10% Other		

Investigations
Confirm ovulation In a menstruating woman, the diagnosis is based on a midluteal (i.e. *1 week before the next period*) serum progesterone > 30 nmol/l, or a urine pregnandiol > 0.5 mmol/ml (samples can be collected weekly). If there is no ovulation in a young woman with no history to suggest PID or endometriosis, it may be worth undertaking ovulation induction for 4 months prior to confirming tubal patency (providing the semen analysis of her partner is normal). If there is anovulation, check early follicular Prl, LH, FSH, T_4, TSH and testosterone. Also check rubella antibodies and, if negative, immunize and advise contraception for 3 months before rechecking serology.

Confirmation of tubal patency This may be by laparoscopy and dye insufflation of the fallopian tubes or by hysterosalpingography. The patient must not be pregnant. Laparoscopy allows exclusion of PID and endometriosis, and avascular peritubal adhesions may be divided (the treatment of vascular adhesions gives poor results).
Salpingostomy for tubal blockage carries conception rates little more than ≈ 20% and IVF may be more appropriate. Tubal surgery should probably be carried out in a specialist centre, if at all.

Male factor infertility
History
This should include alcohol, smoking, sexual development, surgery (particularly maldescent, hernias, varicocele or prostate), urinary problems (? structural abnormality), orchitis (including mumps), recent systemic infections (may temporarily lower the sperm count) and occupation (exposure to toxins). Erectile function, difficulty with penetration and difficulty with ejaculation should also be considered (e.g. IDDM, MS, drugs).

Examination
Carry out a general medical examination, looking particularly at secondary sexual characteristics. In the urogenital examination, look for inguinal scars and check the urethral orifice. Assess the site and size of the testis, confirm the presence of the vas and exclude varicocele or epididymal cysts.

Investigations
Semen analysis varies widely from one ejaculate to another, and two results should be sought at least 1 month apart. Samples should be kept warm in the patient's pocket and brought to the laboratory within 1–2 hours. A 'normal' semen analysis is not proof of ability to fertilize

TABLE 7.12 WHO criteria for normal semen analysis			
Volume:	> 2 ml	Morphology:	> 40% normal
pH:	7–8	Alive:	> 50%
Concentration:	> 20 × 10⁶/ml	WCC:	<1 × 10⁶
Motility:	> 50% forward > 25% with rapid linear progress	Anti-sperm antibodies (MAR test)	Negative

an ovum. See Table 7.12 for the WHO criteria for 'normal' semen analysis.

If the semen analysis is abnormal check LH, FSH, Prl, testosterone and antisperm antibodies. Advise wearing loose-fitting underwear and recheck in 12 weeks. Additional investigations include in vitro tests of sperm–mucus interaction. The postcoital test is not recommended in the routine investigation of infertility, but may be of value if there are real doubts about coital function. Intrauterine insemination is only of value when combined with superovulation, but the increase in the pregnancy rate remains low.

Azoospermia If the FSH is increased there is testicular failure. Check chromosomes. If the FSH is normal there is an obstruction. Is the vas present? (It is absent in cystic fibrosis.) If present, consider scrotal exploration and microsurgical repair. Testicular biopsy will allow recovery of sufficient spermatozoa for ICSI in > 50% of men, even those with elevated FSH.

Oligospermia, teratospermia (abnormal morphology) or asthenospermia (poor motility) Specific causes are rare. Review the history of alcohol, drugs, etc. If a varicocele is present, consider referral to radiologists for embolization, as varicocele treatment improves sperm quality and probably pregnancy rates in oligospermia.

Specific endocrine causes Hyperprolactinaemia usually causes loss of libido (see p. 247). Hypogonadotrophic hypogonadism (low LH, FSH and testosterone) responds well to a GnRH pump or LH + FSH by injection.

Both partners

If investigations of both the man and the woman are normal, the couple should be reviewed. If they are young and have been trying for a relatively short time (e.g. 2 years), it is appropriate to reassure them and adopt a 'wait and see policy' (60–70% of couples will conceive spontaneously in the following 2 years). In unexplained infertility, assisted reproduction may be appropriate after 3–4 years, although perhaps earlier if age is a factor. Ovarian stimulation with intrauterine insemination may also be of benefit in this group. Treatment with clomiphene is not warranted in unexplained infertility.

OVULATION INDUCTION

In a menstruating woman, the diagnosis of ovulation is based on a midluteal (i.e. *1 week before the next period*) serum progesterone > 30 nmol/l or a urine pregnandiol > 0.5 mmol/ml. If the patient has amenorrhoea, exclude pregnancy and give Provera 5 mg TID for 5 days (or gestodene 100 mg IM stat.). If there is a withdrawal bleed use antioestrogens. If there is no bleed, gonadotrophin injections or pulsatile GnRH may be indicated.

Antioestrogens These compete with natural oestrogens by blocking receptors in the pituitary, leading to increased FSH levels. Clomiphene (Clomid) is the initial drug of choice, beginning at 25–50 mg/day PO from days 3–7 of the cycle. The incidence of multiple pregnancy is ≈ 10%. Other side-effects are rare, but include visual disturbances (an indication for withdrawal), hot flushes, breast tenderness, abdominal discomfort and rashes (there have been recent concerns about an increase in the risk of ovarian cancer when clomiphene is used for more than 12 cycles, but this association remains uncertain). Ovarian hyperstimulation is rare, and usually resolves spontaneously. Check a 21-day progesterone level or track weekly urine samples to look for evidence of ovulation.

If there is a spontaneous bleed beginning around days 28–35 the clomiphene should be restarted again for 5 days, again beginning on day 3. If there has been no bleed by day 42, exclude pregnancy and give Provera 10 mg PO BD for 5 days. A withdrawal bleed should be expected within a few days of stopping Provera, and clomiphene again restarted as above. If there has been no ovulation after 2 cycles on 50 mg/day it is reasonable to increase the dose to 100 mg/day PO over the same 5 days for 2 months, then 150 mg for a further 2 months to a maximum 200 mg/day. Failure of oral treatment suggests the need for gonadotrophin therapy. Laparoscopic ovarian drilling with either diathermy or laser is an effective treatment for anovulation in women with clomiphene-resistant PCOS.

Metformin Evidence suggests that metformin 500 mg TID, an oral antidiabetic drug, which works by increasing peripheral utilization of glucose in the presence of endogenous insulin, may also be of value in helping induce ovulation in patients with PCOS (BMJ 2003;951).

Gonadotrophin therapy This should only be carried out with very careful monitoring. Low-dose gonadotrophin injections may be started within a few days of a bleed in a menstruating woman or at any time in amenorrhoea. Injections are given daily and follicle stimulation monitored with USS and serum oestradiol. When one follicle is > 16 mm, hCG is given and the couple advised to have intercourse. Luteal support with hCG is not required (and increases the risk of multiple pregnancy and ovarian hyperstimulation syndrome if given). If initial gonadotrophins are normal or elevated, it may be useful to suppress the HPO axis with an IM or intranasal GnRH analogue before treatment. The multiple pregnancy rate is 20–30% and there is a significant risk of hyperstimulation. Many of these women have PCOS and there is a high spontaneous miscarriage rate ($\approx$ 30%). Purified or recombinant FSH has advantages over older hMG preparations.

Pulsatile GnRH analogue This is a pulsatile SC (or IV) infusion of GnRH by a miniaturized automatic infusion system. Treatment is monitored using ultrasound measurement of follicular development. After ovulation, the pulsatile infusion may be discontinued and luteal support provided. This is a very effective treatment in hypogonadotrophic hypogonadism and usually results in the development of a single follicle.

Hyperstimulation

Ovarian hyperstimulation syndrome is an iatrogenic complication of ovulation induction, usually associated with gonadotrophin use (Table 7.13). It is reported to occur in 0.6–14% of IVF cycles and is characterized by increased vascular permeability, which can lead to fluid in the serous cavities (usually ascites, occasionally pleural and

TABLE 7.13 Classification of ovarian hyperstimulation syndrome

Mild	Moderate	Severe	Critical
Abdominal bloating, mild pain	Increased pain, nausea, diarrhoea	Clinical ascites Haemoconcentration (Hct > 45%, WBC > 15 000/ml)	Tense ascites (Hct > 55%, WBC > 25 000/ml)
Ovarian size usually < 8 cm	Ovarian size usually 8–12 cm with ascites	Oliguria with normal creatinine Liver dysfunction Ovarian size usually < 12 cm	Renal failure Thromboembolic phenomena

rarely pericardial effusion). It tends to be more prolonged and severe if pregnancy occurs, but is nonetheless self-limiting. Fatalities occur.

Treatment

- Liaise with the assisted conception unit.
- Check U&E, FBC (increased haematocrit), LFTs, albumin and clotting. Arrange a USS of the ovaries; look also for ascites.
- Analgesia with paracetamol or with opiates if required.
- Push oral fluids to avoid haemoconcentration. Aim to maintain blood volume and urine output, if necessary using IV crystalloid (normal saline). If haemoconcentration is severe (> 44%) consider colloid ± CVP monitoring.
- Prevent thromboses with support stockings and SC heparin.
- Abdominal paracentesis is practised aggressively by some and gives good symptomatic relief, but it will accentuate the protein loss. It will relieve respiratory compromise and is occasionally useful if oliguria is secondary to pressure of tense ascites on the renal veins.
- The most serious cases may also require drainage of effusions and a dopamine infusion to maintain renal function.
- Surgery should only be undertaken for a ruptured cyst or haemorrhage and by a very experienced operator. TOP may very rarely be required.

ASSISTED REPRODUCTION

Entry guidelines to assisted reproduction units vary, but an example would be: a clear positive recommendation from the GP in a couple with no more than one previous child in a continuing heterosexual relationship of at least 2 years' duration. The woman should be < 40 years old and in good health. (There is no legal requirement for any of these factors.) The couple should be aware of the emotional strain involved. The success rate (i.e. 'take home baby rate' for IVF is ≈ 20%). The incidence of spontaneous miscarriage is increased, as are the risks of multiple pregnancy (≈ 25%), bleeding in pregnancy, PIH (? because of the older population), preterm labour (may be iatrogenic) and SFD neonates. There is no increase in the incidence of congenital abnormality.

IVF

This may be indicated for tubal disease, unexplained infertility, endometriosis, male factor infertility, failed donor insemination or cervical hostility. Donor oocytes may be used with failed ovaries (e.g. Turner syndrome, premature menopause). 'Superovulation' is used for oocyte harvest (Fig. 7.7). HPO down-regulation is achieved initially with GnRH analogues (IM or intranasally) and is followed by FSH in much larger doses than are used for ovulation induction. An injection of hCG (which acts like LH) is given when there are > 3 follicles > 16 mm in diameter. Oocyte retrieval 32–34 hours later is usually carried out transvaginally under systemic sedation using ultrasound-guided needle aspiration (although laparoscopy may be used). Approximately 10% of cycles are abandoned before oocyte harvest, usually in older patients or in those with endometriosis, because of poor ovarian response. Cycles may also be cancelled because of hyperstimulation.

Spermatozoa are prepared and added to the oocyte. At 48 hours after oocyte recovery, a fine plastic cannula is used to place a maximum of three (ideally ≤ 2) embryos 1 cm from the uterine fundus. 'Surplus' embryos can be cryopreserved and replaced 2 days after ovulation in a natural cycle. Luteal support is usually given in IVF or embryo transfer cycles.

ICSI (intracytoplasmic sperm injection)
This involves the in vitro injection of a sperm into an oocyte. The advantages are that any type of sperm (sperm head, immotile sperm, defective sperm) can be injected and that both capacitation and acrosome reaction are unnecessary for fertilization. Sperm can be

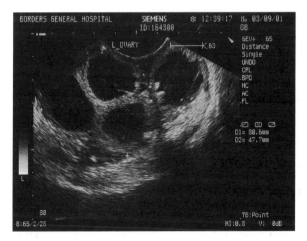

Fig. 7.7 Multiple follicles during hyperstimulation for IVF.

harvested from the epididymis or testis and very small numbers of sperm have been used successfully. Although this technique requires advanced embryological techniques, it has revolutionized the treatment of severe male factor infertility. It is associated with a very small risk of sex chromosome abnormalities and the long-term risks (e.g. infertility in male offspring) are uncertain.

MENOPAUSE

> **The average age at onset of the menopause in the UK is 51 years and is unaffected by parity, age at menarche, or use of the COC but it occurs 6–18 months earlier in smokers. Anovulatory cycles and luteal inadequacy are more common after 40 years of age and may lead to DUB ± endometrial hyperplasia. (See also 'premature ovarian failure', p. 280.)**

Clinical features
Approximately 30% of women are not appreciably affected by flushing or sweating, while these vasomotor symptoms are mild or moderate in ≥ 30% and severe in the remaining ≥ 30%. Seventy-five per cent experience flushing or sweating for more than 1 year and 25% for more than 5 years. Vasomotor symptoms can last from 1 minute to 1 hour and be associated with panic attacks, fatigue and insomnia. Menstrual irregularity is common. Decreased genital blood supply and genital atrophy occur, with loss of hair, elasticity and muscle tone. Vaginal moisture and lubrication are reduced. Anxiety, irritability and depression may be more common after the menopause and libido may decrease.

Longer-term problems may arise, with loss of skin thickness and loss of the cardioprotective effect of oestrogens. There is rapid bone loss for a few years after the menopause and osteoporosis may result. Men have 20% more bone at peak skeletal maturity and fractures are eight times commoner (age for age) than in men.

Diagnosis
Symptoms of the menopause may be mistaken for PMS, depression, thyroid dysfunction, pregnancy and, rarely, phaeochromocytoma or carcinoid syndrome. Hyperprolactinaemia should be excluded, especially in younger women. Vasomotor symptoms may also be caused by calcium antagonists and by antidepressant therapy, especially tricyclics.

Postmenopausally the FSH should be > 30 U/l, but perimenopausally the level may be normal. The physiological midcycle peak of FSH and early-cycle low oestradiol may cause confusion in a premenopausal woman. If there is diagnostic doubt, especially over 45 years of age, a therapeutic trial of HRT may be undertaken. Absence of a satisfactory response suggests that symptoms may not be genuinely menopausal.

Hormone replacement therapy

This involves oestrogen supplementation by oral tablets, transdermal patches, or subcutaneous implants. Daily nasal sprays, skin creams and 3-monthly vaginal rings are also used. Regardless of the route of administration, women who have not undergone hysterectomy should be prescribed a progestogen to reduce the risk of endometrial cancer associated with unopposed oestrogen therapy. This advice applies also to women who have undergone endometrial resection or ablation.

HRT improves vasomotor flushes, sweats, mood problems and vaginal dryness in most patients. It also leads to a significant reduction in osteoporosis and in some fractures. Current evidence indicates, however, that HRT increases the risk of breast cancer, coronary heart disease, stroke and venous thromboembolism, particularly in those using combined oestrogen-progestogen preparations (JAMA 2002;288:321 and Lancet 2003;316:419). Hormone replacement therapy improves short-term symptoms but is (on average) detrimental to future health (BMJ 2004:357). Treatment should therefore be on an informed individualized basis, with risks and benefits carefully considered.

Oral preparations Cyclical combined preparations, which usually lead to monthly withdrawal bleeds, are used perimenopausally, and the continuous combined preparations, the so called 'no-bleed' HRT, are an option from more than 1–2 years after the last menstrual period. Continuous combined therapy is more convenient for the 80–90% who do not experience unscheduled bleeding, but erratic bleeding beyond the first 6–12 months of treatment warrants further investigation.

Alternatives to these oestrogen-progesterone preparations are tibolone and raloxifene. Tibolone is a synthetic steroid with weak oestrogenic, progestogenic and androgenic effects which may be started 2 years after periods have ceased in a similar way to the continuous combined preparations. Raloxifene, a synthetic selective oestrogen-receptor modulator (SERM), has oestrogenic effects on bone but has a minimal effect on uterine and breast tissue (N Engl J Med 1997:1641). It is not effective in controlling perimenopausal symptoms but has a role in protecting against osteoporosis and it does not lead to vaginal bleeding.

Transcutaneous administration Transdermal patches are available as an unopposed oestrogen form, or as cyclical or continuous oestrogen-progestogen combinations. Skin reactions, ranging from hyperaemia to blisters, affect only a small percentage of users. Patches are usually applied to the buttock, and each patch lasts for between 3 and 7 days depending on the formulation. This method appears to be as effective as oral preparations in treating symptomatic women and for the prevention of osteoporosis.

Percutaneous oestrogen gels are also available. A measured dose is rubbed into the skin and avoids the prolonged skin contact of patches. The same contraindications apply as for other unopposed oestrogens.

Subcutaneous implants Oestradiol may be implanted in subcutaneous fat, usually lower abdominally, administering 25–50 mg at intervals of no less than 5–6 months. There is a danger of tachyphylaxis with ever-increasing oestradiol levels and persistent symptoms if strict control of dose is not observed. Monitor preimplant oestradiol levels aiming for < 300–600 pmol/l. Testosterone implants (100 mg) may be used to increase energy and libido although the evidence for this is limited.

Vaginal preparations Tablets of oestradiol, low-dose oestradiol releasing silastic ring pessaries and oestriol vaginal pessaries or vaginal cream may be employed for atrophic vaginitis or trigonitis.

MENORRHAGIA AND DYSMENORRHOEA

> **The menstrual cycle is at its most regular between 20 and 40 years of age, with a tendency towards a longer cycle after menarche and a shorter one before the menopause. The mean menstrual blood loss in the healthy European population is ≈ 40 ml with 70% lost in the first 48 hours. Only 10% lose more than 80 ml (60% of these women become anaemic). The actual blood loss correlates poorly with symptoms, although clotting and flooding are suggestive of heavy bleeding.**

Causes of menorrhagia

1. Uterine pathology – common.
   — Fibroids: 50% of those with menstrual loss > 200 ml have fibroids.
   — Foreign body: e.g. non-progestogen secreting IUCD.
   — The role of PID and polyps is unclear.

2. Dysfunctional uterine bleeding (i.e. no identifiable pelvic pathology) – common.
   — This is the eventual diagnosis in the majority of cases (DUB). The cycles may be anovulatory or ovulatory, but this is of limited clinical importance unless fertility is an issue.
3. Medical disorders – rare.
   — These include hypothyroidism, Cushing's syndrome, bleeding disorders (e.g. von Willebrand's disease or thrombocytopenia, but usually not in women on warfarin or heparin or with coagulation disorders).

Classification of dysmenorrhoea
This may be:

- *Primary (i.e. idiopathic)*: this often occurs in the teenage years and may be related to elevated endometrial production of PGF-2α. Prescribing the COC is frequently of benefit.
- *Secondary*: to fibroids, the IUCD, PID, endometriosis or adenomyosis.

Investigations
A history (including drugs and thyroid symptoms) and clinical examination. It is also important to assess the effects on lifestyle and general well-being. Check a FBC (TFTs only if symptomatic; no other endocrine tests are necessary). Endometrial assessment (see p. 274) should be undertaken in those > 40 years if the periods are irregular or if there has been a recent change in the menses. The risk of endometrial malignancy in women < 40 years old is between 1 : 10 000 and 1 : 100 000, rising to approximately 1 : 100 premenopausally.

Medical treatment
PG synthesis inhibitors. For example, mefanamic acid (Ponstan) 500 mg TID taken at the time of bleeding reduces the mean blood loss by 20–40% in those with menorrhagia. It is also useful for dysmenorrhea. *Side-effects*: 50% have GI problems and 20% experience dizziness or headaches.

Antifibrinolytics For example, tranexamic acid (Cyclokapron) 1 g BD to QID during the time of bleeding reduces mean blood loss by 50% in those with DUB or IUCD-related menorrhagia. *Side-effects*: nausea, vomiting, tinnitus, rash and abdominal cramps. *Contraindications*: a history of thromboembolic disease.

Progestogens For example, medroxyprogesterone acetate (Provera) 5 mg TID on days 5–24 reduces blood loss in DUB (even if the cycles are regular). It is likely that 5 mg TID on days 16–24 has no benefit in those with regular cycles. *Side-effects*: oedema, bloating and weight gain, as well as androgenic problems. Use additional contraception.

COCs These are useful, particularly in younger, non-smoking patients, reducing blood loss by ≈ 50%. They may also be used continuously, e.g. two or three packets may be run together making periods less frequent.

Levonorgestrel impregnated IUCD (Mirena) This acts locally within the uterus to prevent proliferation of the endometrium, and reduces menstrual loss by an average of 90% after 3 months' treatment. Initial worsening of symptoms is common and intermenstrual bleeding occurs frequently, but these problems often settle 5 or 6 months after insertion. Twenty per cent of women experience complete amenorrhoea. Side-effects of lower abdominal discomfort (≈ 10%), skin problems (≈ 5%), and mastalgia (≈ 4%) have been reported, but these figures have not been compared to a control group. There is no change in weight or blood pressure. Mirena has a contraceptive licence for 5 years in the UK; there is good evidence that it remains effective in menstrual dysfunction for up to 7 or 8 years.

Danazol (Danol) This is of no use if taken cyclically. Start with 200 mg/day on a continuous basis. It reduces blood loss, but it may be necessary to increase to 200 mg BD or TID if amenorrhoea is required. *Side-effects*: weight gain, acne, hirsutism, cramps, headaches and breast atrophy (if severe). Use additional contraception.

Surgical treatment

Endometrial ablation All techniques are reported to have good short-term results with ≈ 80% satisfied at 1 year, although amenorrhoea occurs in around a third. There are a number of possible operations, and all are only suitable for those who have completed their families (Table 7.14). The operation is not in itself a contraceptive and pregnancy following the operation carries a high complication rate. Effective contraception is therefore essential and sterilization (male or female) is to be recommended.

Abdominal and vaginal hysterectomy See page 292.

TABLE 7.14 Methods of endometrial ablation

Method	Involves	Advantages and disadvantages
First generation		
TCRE (transcervical endometrial resection) ± rollerball	Direct hysteroscopic vision is used to ablate the endometrium using cutting diathermy ± rollerball	The technique is relatively difficult to learn. Risk of fluid overload and significant risk of damage to surrounding structures
Laser (Nd-YAG)	Direct hysteroscopic vision is used to ablate the endometrium using laser	The technique is also relatively difficult to learn and again carries risks of fluid overload
Second generation		
MEA (microwave endometrial ablation)	Microwaves delivered from intrauterine system	Effective and easy to carry out. Small chance of damage to surrounding structures
Heated balloon system	Ablation with a heated intrauterine water-filled balloon	Very safe, and effective

SPONTANEOUS MISCARRIAGE

Spontaneous miscarriage is the loss of a pregnancy before 24 weeks' gestation. It is most common in the first trimester, with quoted incidences varying from 15% to above 50% depending on the gestation assessed. The word 'abortion' has connotations of induced abortion and should not be used for miscarriage. The term 'blighted ovum' should be discarded in preference to anembryonic pregnancy.

Miscarriage is an important cause of morbidity and even mortality, especially in developing countries, through haemorrhage and infection. Emotional responses include emotional numbness, denial, anxiety, shock, feeling of loss, sadness, emptiness, anger, inadequacy, depression and sleep disturbance. Women experiencing miscarriage are vulnerable and should be cared for with sensitivity and sympathy.

- Congenital uterine abnormalities, see p. 231.
- Fibroids: of uncertain significance, but large fibroids may be a cause of infertility and possibly miscarriage.

Other Although inadequate luteal support may be a cause of miscarriage, there has been no proven benefit from the use of progestogens or hCG. A higher LH level, as in PCOS, is also associated with recurrent miscarriage, but no effective treatment is available. It is also possible that mothers who share a high proportion of HLA antibodies with their partner fail to produce sufficient 'immune blocking antibodies' to protect the fetus from the mother's immune system. Injecting the mother with paternal white cells has not been shown to be effective. Miscarriage is also more likely in association with medical disorders (e.g. renal failure, thyroid dysfunction), although investigation for these is almost always normal.

POSTMENOPAUSAL BLEEDING

> **Postmenopausal bleeding is defined as bleeding from the genital tract 1 year following cessation of the menses. Up to 10% of women with PMB have a primary or secondary malignancy, most commonly endometrial cancer (80%), cervical cancer or an ovarian tumour. Over 90%, therefore, have a benign cause – usually genital tract atrophy and less commonly polyps, endometrial hyperplasia or extragenital pathology.**

Investigations

Whether hysteroscopy or ultrasound, combined with endometrial sampling, is used depends on patient risk factors and local facilities. Pathology can be missed by any of these methods (*www.sign.ac.uk*).

Dilatation and curettage Used alone this will miss 15% of endometrial cancers.

Hysteroscopy This will miss significant pathology in only 3% of cases. It can be carried out either as an inpatient or an outpatient.

Endometrial biopsy The pipelle and the vabra aspirator are the most commonly used tools in the UK. They are both 3 mm in diameter, the pipelle being a thin plastic tube and the vabra a stainless-steel device used with an electrical suction pump. The pipelle is the most convenient, best tolerated and least expensive, but samples only around 4% of the endometrial surface and has a sensitivity of 67–97%

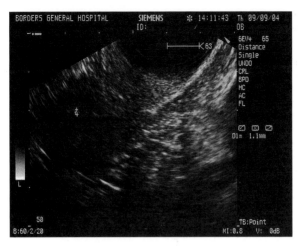

Fig. 7.10 Endometrial carcinoma is very unlikely if the endometrial thickness is less than 4 mm.

for endometrial carcinoma. The vabra samples around 40% of the endometrial surface but is more painful and more expensive. Endometrial biopsy alone is not an adequate method for excluding endometrial malignancy in higher risk groups.

Ultrasound transvaginal scanning This can be used to measure the double layer of endometrial thickness. Endometrial cancer is very unlikely in a postmenopausal woman if the endometrium measures ≤ 4 mm, or ≤ 5 mm for a woman on HRT (Fig. 7.10).

PREMENSTRUAL SYNDROME (PMS)

> **The incidence is 5–95% depending on the criteria used. It occurs more commonly in the multiparous woman, often after the first child. Severe cases are known as premenstrual dysphoric disorder – PMDD**

Symptoms
More than 150 symptoms have been described. The character of the symptoms per se is not so important, but they:

- should occur premenstrually
- should be cyclical
- should disappear or lessen after the onset of menstruation.

Management

- Use a symptom calendar over 3 months to establish the cyclical nature of the symptoms (and therefore the diagnosis).
- Consider other possibilities including major psychiatric disorders (especially bipolar illness), psychosexual problems, endometriosis, PID, PCOS, anaemia, thyroid dysfunction and the menopause (therefore consider Hb, TFTs, FSH).
- If there is serious diagnostic doubt, give a GnRH analogue for 3 months ± continuous combined HRT. Ignore symptoms in the first month, but any symptoms in the third month cannot be attributed to PMS.

Treatment

There may be a significant placebo effect – up to 40% – with many treatments.

- Explanation and reassurance that this is a common condition and that there is no underlying pathology.
- There is now robust evidence to support the use of SSRIs, with most work being carried out using fluoxetine (Prozac) at a dose of 20 mg/day. This is significantly superior to placebo in reducing symptomatology in those with severe PMS if taken on a continuous basis, or in the second half of the cycle (*www.cochrane.co.uk* 2004). The manufacturers have recently been forced to drop PMS from the Prozac indications because of concerns that 'PMDD is not a well-established disease entity across Europe'.
- There is good evidence that Vitamin E, evening primrose oil and progestogens are ineffective in treating PMS and there are, at best, limited data for the use of Vitamin B_6 (pyridoxine).
- The use of the combined oral contraceptive pill for the treatment of PMS is common but there is little support for its efficacy. Some work suggests an improvement in symptoms, whereas other work suggests that those with PMS experience symptom exacerbation.
- GnRH analogues are a highly effective way of suppressing ovarian function, and are therefore a highly effective treatment for severe PMS. As oestrogen is suppressed to postmenopausal levels, however, the PMS symptoms may be replaced by menopausal ones including hot flushes. These in turn can be minimized with the use

of continuous combined 'add-back' HRT. Treatment with GnRH analogues cannot be continued long-term, however, because of the risks of osteoporosis and other side-effects associated with a premature menopause. GnRH analogues are also expensive but there use can be justified not only to demonstrate the potential value of surgery (below) but also as a way of testing the ability to tolerate HRT.

- Bilateral oophorectomy is also a highly effective treatment for PMS. It is, however, a surgical procedure and therefore not without short term surgical risks, even if carried out laparoscopically. More importantly, there are the longer-term risks of premature menopause, particularly if compliance with subsequent HRT is poor. This surgical option is therefore only suitable for those very likely to benefit from it, as suggested by a definite response to a GnRH analogue, and only in those who have completed their family. It is also reasonable not to opt for this procedure if the natural menopause is likely to be occurring relatively soon, and also not to consider the operation in somebody young.

- Some women find self-help groups supportive. General health measures (e.g. improved diet, reducing smoking and drinking, increased exercise, self-relaxation) often help. Herbal remedies are not scientifically tested, but some find them helpful (e.g. sage and fennel for irritability; rosemary, camomile and dandelion for breast tenderness). Some women may also benefit from yoga, hypnosis, homeopathy or acupuncture.

PROLAPSE

Cystourethrocele is the most common prolapse, followed by uterine descent and rectocele. A urethrocele occurring on its own is rare. An enterocele is more common following abdominal hysterectomy, vaginal hysterectomy or colposuspension. Symptoms do not necessarily depend on the size of the prolapse. Treatment may be conservative or surgical (Fig. 7.11).

Conservative treatment
Pelvic floor exercises are useful for minor degrees of prolapse, especially in young women. Pessaries are useful in those who are pregnant, or as a therapeutic test to confirm that surgery would be of

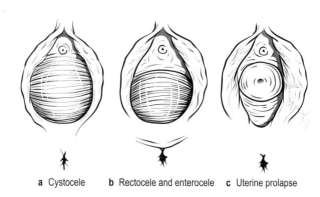

a Cystocele   **b** Rectocele and enterocele   **c** Uterine prolapse

Fig. 7.11 Vaginal prolapse.

benefit, or in those unfit or unwilling to undergo surgery. Ring pessaries are made of inert plastic and will give good vaginal wall support providing that the perineum is sufficiently firm posteriorly to hold the ring in situ. The ring rests in the posterior fornix and sits over the symphysis pubis anteriorly (if fitting a ring on the first occasion, choose one with a diameter approximately equal to the posterior fornix–symphysis distance as estimated by a digital examination). A shelf-pessary is useful for uterine prolapse. Rings should be removed every 6–12 months, the vault inspected for inflammation or ulceration, and a new ring replaced. Short courses of topical vaginal oestrogens are occasionally required.

Surgical treatment

Cystocele Prolapse of the bladder (± urethra) may lead to discomfort, the feeling of 'something coming down' or urinary symptoms, particularly stress incontinence. Urgency and frequency are associated with cystocele and may (but do not necessarily) improve following surgery. A cystocele may also rarely cause obstruction, leading to urinary retention and overflow incontinence. Surgical correction of cystocele may be by anterior colporrhaphy (anterior repair) in which the vaginal skin is divided in the midline, the bladder (and urethra if there is a urethrocele) reflected upwards and the pubocervical fascia on either side buttressed with interrupted sutures. Redundant vaginal skin is excised and the vaginal epithelium closed. Postoperative urinary retention is uncommon, but may justify the use of a urethral or suprapubic catheter. Burch colposuspension will also correct a cystocele and is more effective in improving stress incontinence (see p. 303).

Uterus and cervix This may cause low backache, often relieved by lying flat. It is graded as first degree (there is some descent within the vagina), second degree (the cervix appears at the introitus) or third degree (or procidentia , i.e. the uterus is completely outside the vagina). With a procidentia, there may be ulceration, bleeding or an offensive discharge. Correction is by vaginal hysterectomy ± anterior or posterior repair. A Manchester repair (cervical amputation with anterior and posterior repair) probably also has a role in first- and second-degree prolapse.

Enterocele (herniation of the Pouch of Douglas) and vault prolapse These contain peritoneum and usually the small bowel or omentum. Enteroceles are repaired by opening the vaginal wall in the midline and dissecting the enterocele so that it is free, ligating it and closing the vaginal wall. Vault prolapse (after hysterectomy) is traditionally treated by an abdominal colposacropexy (a non-absorbable mesh is used to join the vault to the anterior longitudinal ligament over the first sacral vertebra), but may be more easily managed with a vaginal sacrospinous ligament fixation (the vault is supported by a stitch through the sacrospinous ligament, usually on just one side). This latter procedure probably carries a higher failure rate but less morbidity.

Rectocele This may give rise to backache, a lump in the vagina and a feeling of incomplete bowel emptying. The patient may be having to press the rectocele upwards at the time of defecation, or may be having to use digital evacuation. A vertical posterior vaginal wall incision is used to dissect the levator ani muscles and rectum. The levator ani muscles are sutured to the superficial perineal muscles, the redundant vaginal skin excised and the incision closed. It is easy to leave the vagina too narrow, and therefore only a little skin should be excised.

SECONDARY AMENORRHOEA

> **This is defined as no menstruation for 6 months (or > three times the previous cycle length) in the absence of pregnancy.**

The commonest causes are PCOS, weight loss, hyperprolactinaemia.

Initial management

- Exclude pregnancy.
- Ask about perimenopausal symptoms (e.g. flushings, vaginal dryness).
- Take a history, including weight changes, drugs, medical disorders and thyroid symptoms.
- Carry out an examination looking particularly at height, weight, visual fields and the presence of hirsutism or virilization. Consider carrying out a pelvic examination.
- Check serum for LH, FSH, Prl, testosterone, T_4 and TSH.
- Arrange a transvaginal USS; look for polycystic ovaries.
- Review back in the clinic with the results.

Further management

Ultrasound scan A scan showing multiple (> 8) small, peripherally placed follicular ovarian cysts surrounded by a thickened echodense stroma confirms the diagnosis of polycystic ovaries. The diagnosis is supported by an LH : FSH ratio > 3 and a testosterone level > 3 mmol/l (see PCOS, p. 244).

Elevated prolactin level The Prl is > 800 mU/l on at least two occasions (see hyperprolactinaemia, p. 247).

Elevated FSH (> 30 U/l) Repeat the sample 6 weeks later. If FSH is still elevated and the patient > 40 years old, the patient is menopausal (see p. 264). If the patient is < 40 years old, the diagnosis is premature ovarian failure. This occurs in 1% of women and may be due to viral infections (e.g. mumps), cytotoxic drugs or radiotherapy. It is most commonly idiopathic, and is only occasionally associated with chromosomal abnormality (XO mosaics or XXX). A low oestrogen level, very high FSH and the absence of any menstrual activity are poor prognostic signs for recovery. An ovarian biopsy is generally not indicated, as the histological correlation with prognosis is poor. Treat with HRT. Pregnancy by IVF with donor oocytes is possible. There is an association with other autoimmune disorders, so check antiovarian antibodies, FBC (? pernicious anaemia) and thyroid function.

Abnormal TFTs If the TFTs are abnormal, treat as appropriate.

If the above tests are normal, consider the following:

Weight loss The weight usually needs to be more than 45 kg, or the BMI (weight [kg]/height [m^2]) (see Appendix 6) greater than 17 for menstruation to occur. Loss of 10–15% weight usually leads to amenorrhoea. Anorexia nervosa is uncommon, with an incidence probably less than 1%. It can develop prior to menarche, is usually lifelong and is characterized by loss of insight regarding the distorted body image. There is loss of hair, increased lanugo, decreased pulse, lowered BP, anaemia, low basal LH and FSH and low oestrogen. Ovulation induction is possible with clomiphene or pulsatile GnRH in those wishing to conceive, but there is a much increased risk of fetal loss, IUGR and premature labour, so that it is ideal to wait until weight is restored spontaneously. Return of menstrual function may not be until months after the weight has been restored. The prevalence of bulimia is ≈ 1% and of these 60% will have had an episode of amenorrhoea at some time.

Depression, acute emotional disturbance and extreme exercise
These may lead to amenorrhoea.

Sheehan syndrome Necrosis of the anterior pituitary following severe PPH is now very rare in the UK. It presents with failure of lactation, apathy, loss of axillary and pubic hair with symptoms and signs of hypothyroidism and adrenocortical insufficiency.

Asherman syndrome Secondary amenorrhoea following destruction of the endometrium by curettage is also relatively rare. Multiple synechiae are seen at hysteroscopy. Treatment involves breaking down the adhesions through a hysteroscope ± inserting an IUCD to deter reformation.

Idiopathic amenorrhoea This is sometimes called euoestrogenic amenorrhoea and usually responds well to clomiphene if fertility is required.

SEXUAL HEALTH

Sexual dysfunction is a common symptom in the gynaecology clinic, and patients' ability to share their problem often depends on the attitude of the clinician. Simple, open-ended questions asked in a relaxed, non-judgmental atmosphere are appropriate. The possibility of sexual dysfunction should be particularly borne in mind in infertility and colposcopy clinics, after gynaecological surgery (especially for cancer) and in those on medication (anticholinergics, antidepressants, spironolactone, cimetidine, steroids, antihypertensives).

The history should include the problem as the patient sees it, how long the problem has been present and whether the problem is related to the time, place or partner. It is also important to establish whether there is a loss of sex drive or dislike of sexual contact, or whether there are problems within the relationship. Consider whether there is anxiety, guilt or anger that is not being expressed, and enquire about whether there are physical problems (e.g. pain) with either partner. A social history is appropriate and medical history essential (depression, diabetes, osteoarthritis).

It is good practice to offer to have a chaperone present for both male and female patients if they wish. A substantial minority of patients, both men and women, prefer to be examined by a doctor of their own sex (remember that patients have made complaints of indecent assault, even when their examining doctor was of the same sex). Cultural differences must also be considered. Many Muslim, Hindu and Sikh women practise a strict sexual morality. Girls are brought up to be shy and modest, and submitting to a vaginal examination may be regarded with abhorrence, even as a matter of life and death. Remember that your own sexual mores may not be universally accepted.

Examination is necessary when a physical problem is suspected but may not always be appropriate. In the female patient assess the development of secondary sexual characteristics and exclude hirsutism or other signs of virilization. Examine the abdomen and the reflexes, including a check of the anal reflex if a neurological problem is suspected. Digital and speculum examination of the vagina may be appropriate to exclude congenital abnormalities, infection, episiotomy scarring, uterine tenderness and adnexal pathology. Endocrine investigation has a limited role but LH, FSH, T_4, Prl and testosterone may be relevant. Genital and systemic examinations in the male may also be appropriate, looking particularly for gynaecomastia, and testing for tactile (dorsal column) and pinprick (spinothalamic tract) sensation in the perineal and lower limb dermatomes. Check urinalysis for sugar.

Dyspareunia

This is common and may be due to organic pathology. The pain may be reproducible during VE. It may be superficial (e.g. vulvovaginitis, Bartholin's gland cyst, episiotomy scars) or deep (e.g. endometriosis, chronic PID, ovarian cysts, large fibroids, retroverted uterus). Frequently, however, examination (which may include laparoscopy) is normal. Vaginismus, poor lubrication and penetration before arousal are common causes of dyspareunia. There may be help with the use of different sexual positions. If the vagina is dry, a lubricating gel (e.g. KY Jelly) ±HRT perimenopausally may be of help.

Vaginismus

This is characterized by involuntary spasm of the pubococcygeus muscle such that penetration is difficult or impossible. It may begin after a minor episode of pain (e.g. due to thrush) and occur on subsequent occasions before penetration to prevent the painful episode happening again. This makes penetration more painful and so the cycle continues, being further exacerbated by anxiety. Vaginismus may be related to personality, sexual attitudes or the ability to become aroused. Speculum and vaginal examination may be impossible. Vaginismus is best treated by using graded vaginal dilators with regular supervision and encouragement (± sensate focus, see p. 286) and Kegel exercises to allow voluntary relaxation of the pubococcygeus.

Orgasmic dysfunction

This may be associated with general sexual dysfunction. If it occurs despite achieving arousal, it is best managed with instruction in masturbatory techniques.

General sexual dysfunction

This is lack of sexual interest or arousal. It is often associated with guilt, self-blame and at times positive avoidance of sex. Ask about symptoms of depression or anxiety. Remember that breast-feeding is a powerful cause of lack of sex drive (due to high prolactin levels).

Erectile difficulty

Penile erection is due to relaxation of the smooth muscle around the cavernosal vascular spaces, allowing them to fill with blood. This is under the control of the autonomic nervous system, mediated by cyclic guanosine monophosphate (cGMP). Erectile failure is common, with 52% of men aged 40–70 years suffering the problem to some degree. As approximately 75% will have an organic component, drug treatment is now often used in addition to, or instead of, psychosexual counselling.

Treatment options include one of the phosphodiesterase type 5 inhibitors, which are taken orally and act as an enhancer of erection by blocking breakdown of cGMP, e.g. sildenafil (Viagra), tadalafil or vardenafil. They work best in psychogenic erectile failure and milder organic problems in which the success rate is ≈ 85%. Side-effects are mild and transient and include flushing, dyspepsia, headache and transient disturbance in colour vision. It must not be used with nitrates (may lead to a potentially life-threatening profound drop in BP).

Alprostadil (PGE_1) relaxes cavernosal smooth muscle but must be injected directly into the corpora cavernosa. It is more effective than sildenafil in erectile failure due to more severe organic problems. Other treatments include vacuum devices and penile implants, the latter only being suitable where no other treatment has been effective.

Ejaculatory problems

Premature ejaculation may be defined as the tendency to ejaculate too quickly for his own, or his partner's, satisfaction. Delayed ejaculation is the reverse and is more difficult to treat. Retrograde ejaculation occurs when the seminal fluid passes backwards into the bladder (e.g. postprostatectomy, spinal cord injury). A man with premature ejaculation can learn to delay his ejaculation by means of a programme of graded masturbatory exercises (the squeeze technique). Intercourse should proceed as usual until ejaculation is felt to be inevitable. The couple should then stop and either the man or his partner should squeeze just below the glans penis. This is repeated four or five times before ejaculation is allowed to occur. Fluoxetine 20 mg/day on days when intercourse is planned often helps in severe cases.

Reduced sexual desire

As in the female, this is poorly understood, but may be related to upbringing, poor social skills, lack of opportunity or lack of sexual education. Increased Prl is a rare cause, and some men aged > 50 years have decreased testosterone due to testicular failure and may require testosterone replacement.

TREATMENT FOR THE COUPLE

It is important to exclude organic pathology, and laparoscopy may be warranted, particularly in dyspareunia. The routine gynaecology clinic is an inappropriate setting for a series of long consultations (unless at the end of the clinic) and continuity with one counsellor is crucial. Consider referral to a sexual dysfunction clinic. Both partners should attend, as they usually both contribute to the problems.

Management

In some instances, reassurance or information may be all that is required. Patients sometimes want to check that their sexual practice is normal (e.g. positions used, oral sex). This includes confirming that it is acceptable to be less sexually active (e.g. in the puerperium or postmenopausally) or may apply to sexual orientation. Although our society encourages discussion about sexuality, there is still ignorance and naiveté in some couples (e.g. they are unaware that the rate of arousal is faster in males than in females and that penetration before the female is aroused will result in pain from dryness and failure of ballooning of the vagina).

Also note that:

- Most women are more likely to achieve orgasm by masturbation, partner digital stimulation of clitoris or oral sex than by penetrative intercourse.
- Most women do not experience multiple orgasms
- Women may initiate sex.
- Intercourse is not essential (unless fertility is required).
- Masturbation (including using a vibrator) is neither dirty nor harmful.
- If a man loses his erection, it does not mean he does not find his partner attractive.
- Reduced libido is common in pregnancy and the puerperium.

Intensive therapy Dyspareunia (without identifiable cause), the orgasmic dysfunctions and the male dysfunctions may be treated with a behavioural approach (e.g. 12 fortnightly consultations). This treatment (sensate focus, Table 7.15) consists of a programme of tasks that a couple can undertake in their own time at home. Underlying the programme is a ban on sexual intercourse or any genital contact until anxiety about performance and fear of failure have subsided and trust between the couple has been established. This ban ensures that physical intimacy will not lead to sexual intimacy. The tasks involve the couple setting aside time to explore each other's bodies in turn by touching, stroking, caressing and massaging, gradually introducing sensual, then erotic, and then sexual touch over a period of time. About two-thirds will be 'much improved', although there is a significant long-term recurrence rate. Once again, this is best carried out in a specific clinic rather than by generalists in a gynaecology setting.

The couple need to be monitored to agree the ground rules and the staged tasks, to deal with any issues that may arise as a result of the tasks, to support positive changes and prevent relapse in the early stages. Suggested ground rules are:

- Agree a ban on sexual intercourse and genital touching.
- Set up twice-weekly times to spend on this homework, increasing from 20 minutes to 60 minutes over 4 weeks.
- During these times, speak only if the partner's touch is painful or unacceptable. Otherwise it is assumed that what is being done is all right. Conversation will prevent concentration on the task and render it pointless.
- Attention should be focused on personal experience, not on pleasing the partner. This is a learning exercise above all.

TABLE 7.15 Sensate focus

Stage 1

1. Taking plenty of time, each person explores the other's naked (if possible) body, avoiding breasts and genitals, avoiding trying to give pleasure, and concentrating on feelings and sensations experienced in both 'active' and 'passive' roles.
2. After 2 weeks or 4 sessions of this, some familiarity and trust should allow inclusion of breasts and experimentation with a variety of touches, such as with body oils, talcum powder, feathers, fabrics, etc.
3. As above but adding the making of specific requests for preferred types of touch and the use of a back-to-front position to enable the person being touched to guide the partner's hand.

Stage 2

1. Maintain the ban on intercourse, but include genital touching as part of the established exercises, so there are now no forbidden areas.
2. While continuing all the above, concentrate more on the genitals to discover the sensations resulting from different pressures in different areas.
3. This is an optional stage for mutual masturbation to orgasm.

Stage 3

1. While continuing all the above and maintaining the ban on full intercourse, the next step is containment without movement, allowing the penis to be accepted and contained by the vagina (modified for homosexual couples). Couples should progress at their preferred pace.
2. Containment with gentle thrusting and rotating movement.
3. Thrusting to orgasm.

SURGERY IN GYNAECOLOGY

This section is not intended as a surgical textbook but is a guide for those beginning their surgical experience to appreciate the sequence of events in a few selected basic procedures. It is in no way a substitute for experienced practical teaching, and surgery must not be undertaken without appropriate supervision.

PREOPERATIVE CONSIDERATIONS

- Does the patient need the operation? Have alternatives been considered and discussed (e.g. see alternatives to surgery for menorrhagia, p. 267)?
- Make sure the patient is not pregnant.

Consent
See particularly page 336. Some areas of controversy are highlighted below:

Sterilization
See page 226 and ensure that all the points covered have been fully documented.

Hysterectomy
Subtotal hysterectomy carries a lower morbidity than a total abdominal hysterectomy – there is less bleeding and fewer wound and urine infections and a lower incidence of urinary tract damage. Vaginal hysterectomy is probably superior to the abdominal approach in appropriate cases in that there is no abdominal wound and there is also a lower incidence of bladder, ureteric and bowel injury (Table 7.16). Laparoscopically assisted procedures are not discussed here.

Normal ovaries at abdominal hysterectomy
Whether to remove ovaries at abdominal hysterectomy or not depends on the patient's wishes, her age, her family history of breast or ovarian carcinoma (p. 329) and her plans for HRT (p. 265). In someone who is 50 years old, it is unlikely that there will be much further ovarian function (average age of menopause is 51, p. 264), and bilateral salpingo-oophorectomy will greatly reduce the incidence of later ovarian carcinoma. Residual ovaries may also occasionally cause chronic pain or dyspareunia if adherent to the vaginal vault or pelvic side-wall. In someone who is 40, however, a further 10 years of ovarian oestrogen secretion may be expected. It is unclear whether HRT is as effective in terms of long-term prophylaxis as endogenous oestrogens. It may therefore be appropriate to discuss routine oophorectomy in those over 45 and ovarian conservation in those under 45. The decision must remain, however, a very individualized consideration.

Bladder, bowel and sexual dysfunction after hysterectomy
There is conflicting evidence about whether abdominal hysterectomy has any effect on bladder function (there have been no studies looking

TABLE 7.16 Pros and cons of different hysterectomy routes

Methods	Pros	Cons
Total abdominal hysterectomy	Cervix is removed therefore no further smears or risk of cervical malignancy (therefore particularly suitable for those with a history of abnormal cytology) Good access to ovaries	Increased surgical morbidity
Subtotal abdominal hysterectomy	Fewer complications than TAH (↓ bleeding, ↓ infection, ↓ bladder injury, ↓ ureteric damage) Good access to ovaries	Risk of cervical cancer remains as before. Up to 10% will require subsequent removal due to bleeding
Vaginal hysterectomy	Lower incidence of bladder and bowel injury in straightforward cases (compared to abdominal hysterectomy) No potentially painful abdominal wound	There is only limited ovarian access Is contraindicated with: • large uterus • restricted uterine mobility • limited vaginal space • adnexal pathology • cervix flush with vagina

at vaginal hysterectomy and urinary dysfunction). The picture is just as confused with bowel function. With regard to sexual dysfunction it is probable that women who retain an overall normal sexual desire have improved postoperative satisfaction due to relief of presenting symptoms.

Antibiotic prophylaxis

There is evidence that the use of single or short courses of broad spectrum antibiotics at the time of major surgery reduces the incidence of postoperative infection. Screening for chlamydia ± antibiotic prophylaxis for those < 30 years undergoing uterine instrumentation is also appropriate.

Venous thromboembolic prophylaxis

Venous thromboembolic disease accounts for around 20% of perioperative hysterectomy deaths. As prophylaxis is effective in reducing thromboembolism, all gynaecological patients should be assessed for risk factors and prophylaxis prescribed accordingly. The incidence is higher in those with malignancy (35%), lower for 'routine' abdominal hysterectomy (12%) and lowest for vaginal hysterectomy.

As some prophylactic methods may be associated with side-effects (e.g. wound haematomas and hypersensitivity reactions with heparin) the methods chosen must be based on some form of risk vs benefit assessment (Tables 7.17, 7.18). The benefits to the patient of heparin in moderate/high risk groups are felt to outweigh the approximately 2 : 100 risk of wound haematoma, which may be minimized by avoiding injection close to the wound. Graduated compression stockings would be an alternative although compliance with stockings may be reduced in those who find them uncomfortable. In addition, they have not been shown to reduce the risk of fatal pulmonary thromboembolism. Dextran carries a significant risk of anaphylaxis.

Any benefits to stopping the COC 4–6 weeks prior to surgery must be weighed against the risk of unwanted pregnancy. In the absence of other risk factors there is insufficient evidence to support a policy of routine COC discontinuation. HRT probably does not require to be stopped for surgery.

TABLE 7.17 Meta-analysis of incidence of deep venous thrombosis after major general surgery (defined by ^{125}I scanning)

Prophylaxis	Mean incidence (%)
No prophylaxis	25
Low dose heparin	9
Graduated elastic compression stockings	9
Intermittent pneumatic compression	10
Dextran	17
Aspirin	20

SPECIFIC SURGICAL CONSIDERATIONS

Cut well, tie well, get well! (Denton Cooley, pioneering cardiac transplant surgeon)

Assisting and operating

It is important to master good technique at the start, as bad habits are hard to lose. Practise releasing clamps slowly and steadily with each

TABLE 7.18 Risk factors for venous thromboembolic disease (incidences based on BMJ 1992; 305: 567 and suggested prophylaxis based on RCOG Working Party 1995)

Risk group	Details	DVT	Proximal vein thrombosis	Fatal pulmonary embolism	Suggestion for prophylaxis
Low risk groups	Minor surgery (< 30 minutes); no risk factors other than age Major surgery (< 30 minutes); age < 40; no other risk factors (as below)	< 10%	< 1%	0.01%	Early mobilization +/– TED stockings
Moderate risk group	Minor surgery (< 30 minutes) with personal or FH of DVT, PE or thrombophilia Major gynaecological surgery (> 30 minutes) Age > 40 years, obesity (> 80 kg), gross VVs, current infection Immobility prior to surgery (> 4 days) Major medical illness: heart or lung disease, cancer, inflammatory bowel disease	10–40%	1–10%	0.1–1%	Early mobilization + TED stockings + heparin (e.g. 5000 U BD S/C or enoxaparin 20 mg/d)
High risk group	Three or more of above risk factors Major pelvic or abdominal surgery for cancer Major surgery in patients with previous DVT, pulmonary embolism, thrombophilia, or lower limb paralysis (e.g. hemiplegic stroke, paraplegia)	40–80%	10–30%	1–10%	Early mobilization + TED stockings + heparin (e.g. 5000 U TID S/C or enoxaparin 40 mg/d)

hand. Use forceps and scissors with your hands supinated (allows a better view of the end of the instrument). Ask someone who can tie knots properly to show you how, and practise single and double throws, ensuring that each throw is tied in the opposite direction to the one below it. The knots should be tightened with the index or middle fingers pulling in opposite directions (otherwise there is tension on the structure being tied rather than on the knot itself).

Ask for the lights to be arranged to maximal benefit. Stand on two feet, not one. Lean your hips against the table for support (not your elbows on the patient's chest). If making an incision, apply even tension to the skin to allow a cleaner cut. If swabbing out, try not to traumatize visceral structures or tied pedicles, which may make bleeding worse. If there is deep venous bleeding, it is often easier to identify the site using suction rather than swabs. It is well worth reading traditional accounts of the fine points of theatre technique, (e.g. Bonney's Gynaecological Surgery, Cassell, London).

EUA, dilatation and curettage ± hysteroscopy

Place the patient in the lithotomy position. Inspect the vulva. If a smear is required, do this before washing and draping. Carry out a thorough EUA, noting uterine size, shape, mobility and the presence of adnexal masses (it is usually possible to feel normal ovaries unless the patient is obese). Insert a Sims' speculum and grasp the anterior lip of the cervix with at least one volsellum. Check for uterine descent and lateral access (i.e. suitability for vaginal hysterectomy if this is ever required). Insert a uterine sound gently, taking care that the angulation of the curve is in the direction of the uterine cavity (i.e. concave anteriorly for an anteverted uterus) and measure to the cavity length. Beware of creating a false passage or perforating the uterine fundus (it helps to hold a finger on the sound and dilators to prevent sudden slippage). If perforation occurs, abandon the procedure and consider antibiotics. If the uterus was perforated with a sound or small dilator, conservative management is probably appropriate. If perforation was with a suction curette or grasping forceps the risk of bowel injury is much higher, and laparoscopy or laparotomy should be considered.

The extent of dilatation depends on the instrument to be inserted (e.g. 5–6 mm for a 5 mm hysteroscope, 5–10 mm for a curette, and approximately the number of weeks of gestation for TOP or ERPOC, usually 8, 10 or 12 weeks being 8, 10 or 12 mm). A hysteroscope can use fluid (e.g. Hartman's solution) or CO_2 to insufflate the cavity. After inspection of the cavity and both ostia it is common to curette radially to obtain an endometrial sample (e.g. at 10, 2, 5 and 7 o'clock, or at any specific area thought to be suspicious at hysteroscopy). ERPOC or suction TOP up to 12 weeks is best performed with suction through either a flexible or a rigid curette (see p. 298). A balance needs to be struck between excessive curettage, which might lead to Asherman's syndrome, and leaving tissue behind (an empty uterus has a sandpaper feel on curettage).

Laparoscopy

Place the patient in the Lloyd Davis position. Ensure asepsis. Empty the bladder, unless you are certain that the patient has voided just prior to theatre. Instrument the uterus only if you are certain that there is no intrauterine pregnancy. After putting the patient's head downwards, insufflate the abdomen with CO_2. This can either be done blind (Veress needle inserted subumbilically and aimed towards the coccyx to avoid the aortic bifurcation, or suprapubically aimed posteriorly) or under direct vision after cut-down, particularly if there are concerns about adhesions. Check that the flow rate is normal and that the abdomen is distending symmetrically and becoming resonant. After insufflating ≈ 2 litres of gas the needle is removed and a trochar inserted for the telescope ± camera. All subsequent ports should be under direct intra-abdominal vision by telescope. Midline ports have a much lower associated incidence of Richter's herniae and midline entry also minimizes the risk of injury to the inferior epigastric artery (runs from the external iliac artery upwards, anterior to the arcuate ligament and then between the posterior lamina of the rectus sheath and posterior aspect of rectus abdominis). Carry out a thorough inspection of pelvic organs, including lifting the ovaries to check the ovarian fossae. If tubal function is being assessed, inject dilute methylene blue through the cervical cannulae and inspect the fimbrial end of each tube. If PID is suspected, check the liver (? peri-hepatic adhesions, p. 254).

At the end, release the gas. Some clinicians leave ports to heal spontaneously while others suture the skin. Lateral ports > 10 mm carry a high risk of Richter's herniae and should have the sheath and skin closed, care being taken not to include viscera in the stitch (there are a number of specialized techniques for this).

Abdominal hysterectomy

This may be carried out using a lower abdominal transverse incision (as for caesarean section, see p. 119) or, if the uterus is large or there are large ovarian cysts, through a midline or paramedian incision. If malignancy is suspected, take saline washings on opening the peritoneum, and palpate the paracolic gutters, liver and diaphragm. Place two clamps just lateral to the uterus on either side over the round and broad ligaments (Fig. 7.12), taking care to leave the tips well short of the bladder. Angle the tips slightly outwards into the broad ligament

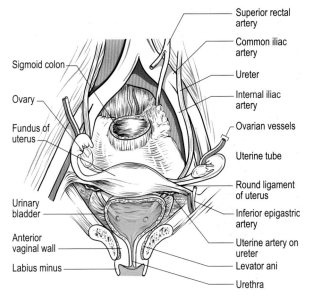

Fig. 7.12 Pelvic anatomy – anterior view.

to avoid cutting the ascending uterine artery just lateral to the uterine body. If taking the ovary, clamp the round ligament laterally and divide it to open up the leaves of the broad ligament. Taking a finger posteriorly, press it through the posterior leaf of the broad ligament lateral to the ovary (i.e. under the infundibulopelvic ligament) and push it up to the space in the divided round ligament. Clamp the infundibulopelvic ligament, taking care that it does not contain the ureter as it crosses the pelvic brim (this is usually a problem only if anatomy is distorted, e.g. by severe endometriosis or a large ovarian cyst). Divide medial to the clamp. This and the lateral part of the round ligament should be tied and may be double tied together for extra security. Repeat on the other side. If the ovaries are not being taken it is usually possible to draw the ovary laterally (one finger in front and the other behind the broad ligament) and place a second clamp medial to the ovary, with the point almost touching the initial clamp. The round and ovarian ligaments can then be divided and tied together.

Open the uterovesical peritoneum by lifting with dissecting forceps and dividing with scissors, starting from the already partially opened broad ligament laterally. This allows the bladder to be pushed downwards, either with a swab or by freeing it with scissors, care being taken to keep the scissor points pointing posteriorly away from the bladder. If in the wrong plane (usually too superficial) there may be a lot of troublesome bleeding from the venous plexus behind the bladder. The lateral angles of the bladder need to be given attention to ensure that the ureters are clear. Also, palpate to ensure that the ureter is out of the way before clamping each uterine artery and ligating the pedicles. Particular care of the ureter is required in the presence of fibroids or endometriosis.

There are many different ways to complete the operation. The top of the vagina may be opened in the midline with a scalpel, cutting laterally with scissors to clamp the cardinal and uterosacral ligaments before continuing round to the back of the vagina. Alternatively, these ligaments can be clamped initially, working downwards to the vaginal vault before opening the vagina to remove the uterus. Throughout, care is necessary to avoid damage to bladder, ureters and bowel. A non-suction drain can be inserted before closure if there are concerns about on-going bleeding. The vault can be closed with an interrupted or continuous suture.

Vaginal hysterectomy

Grasp the cervix (Fig. 7.13) with volsellum forceps and pull down. Circumcise it all the way around, allowing the bladder to be reflected upwards anteriorly (opening the uterovesical pouch at this point if possible). The pouch of Douglas should be visualized posteriorly. Open the pouch with scissors, widen it digitally and clamp the uterosacral ± the cardinal ligaments laterally. Dividing and tying these allows the uterine arteries to be clamped and divided, and access obtained to the broad ligament, round ligament and fallopian tube. These can then also be clamped and divided. Throughout, keep as close into the uterus as possible to avoid injury to more lateral structures. With a larger uterus, or where access is more difficult, it is often necessary to take multiple pedicles on each side rather than the four described. After ensuring haemostasis there are a number of ways to close, but the uterosacral and cardinal ligaments are often sutured into the vault to provide support. The vault itself is then closed with continuous or interrupted sutures.

Anterior colporrhaphy

Grasp the cervix with volsellum forceps and pull down. Consider injecting 10–20 ml of 0.5% bupivacaine with 1 : 200 000 adrenaline superficially to the cystocele to aid haemostasis. Make a small transverse incision above the cervix but below the bladder, and attach two small clips to the upper lip of this. It is then possible to run a pair

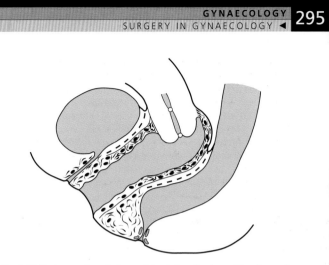

Fig. 7.13 Vagina, cervix and uterus – lateral view. The barred lines (– – – –) define the avascular areolar planes between the thick vascular vaginal walls and the bladder (anteriorly), and the rectum (posteriorly). These planes extend up to the peritoneal reflections. Note: below the bladder neck and the apex of the perineal body, there are no natural planes of separation.

of curved scissors (points upwards) into the relatively avascular plane between the vaginal mucosa and the bladder, allowing division of the mucosa in the midline. This is held laterally while the bladder is reflected, care being taken to ensure that the reflection is started as far laterally as possible to avoid bladder damage and that it is reflected in the avascular plane. The bladder is then pushed well upwards.

Two or three buttressing sutures are placed as deeply as possible into the lateral fascia, redundant skin is excised in the midline and the full thickness of vaginal wall reapposed with interrupted sutures.

Posterior colporrhaphy

Incise the posterior fourchette transversely for 1–2 cm and grasp the upper lip of the incision with two small clips. As for the anterior colporrhaphy, use curved scissors to identify the avascular plane between the vagina and rectum and divide the vaginal skin vertically in the midline. Again, use sharp and blunt dissection to push the bowel laterally, free of the vaginal skin on each side. Buttress the fascia on each side with interrupted sutures before excising redundant skin (take care in posterior vaginal surgery not to excise too much skin) and close with a continuous or interrupted suture. If there is also an enterocele, it is necessary to extend the incision upwards over this, opening the sac of peritoneum, reducing the contents and ligating it as high as possible before reclosing.

Course of the ureter

The ureter runs a retroperitoneal course from the renal pelvis downwards and slightly medially over psoas major, entering the pelvis over the external iliac artery and vein. It runs down over the anterior branch of the internal iliac artery and follows the anterior border of the greater sciatic notch until, opposite the ischial spine, it turns anteromedially into the fascia of the lower part of the broad ligament. It then continues medially towards the cervix. Two centimetres lateral to the cervix it is crossed by the uterine artery before turning anteriorly to the base of the bladder. The uterine artery in turn reaches the side of the uterus and ascends to anastomose with the ovarian artery from above as well as sending branches downwards to the cervix and vagina.

POSTOPERATIVE CONSIDERATIONS

> **Check that thromboprophylactic measures are in place.**

The most likely complication in the first 24 postoperative hours is haemorrhage. If there are significant signs of haemorrhage (blood in drain, pale patient, increased pulse, decreased BP, distending pale abdomen) it may often be necessary to return to theatre. Experienced surgical help should be sought. Site two IV infusions, crossmatch 6 U RCC, check clotting, and involve the anaesthetist early.

In the routine postoperative days, check the patient's general appearance, and look for pyrexia, abdominal pain and distension, and urinary or bowel difficulties. If the haemoglobin has fallen, consider whether the loss in theatre was sufficient to account for the drop, or whether there might be a haematoma (pain, pyrexia, delayed restoration of bowel sounds and, occasionally, urinary retention). management is often conservative unless problems are severe.

If the patient is pyrexial, are there symptoms or signs to suggest UTI, DVT or chest infection? Send an MSU sample for analysis. Note that 50% of DVTs have no demonstrable clinical signs (see DVT management, p. 204). Abdominal distension may be the result of a haematoma (as above), postoperative ileus or true bowel obstruction. Consider AXR if there is possible ileus or bowel obstruction.

Discharge Try and ensure that the patient knows what has been done and why. What, if anything, happens next? What medication has been described and what follow-up is to be arranged (find out who is to make the appointment)? Does the patient need to see the GP? Are there any results still to get? Who should the patient contact if there is a problem? If appropriate, ensure HRT has been started (see p. 265). Also, discuss resumption of activity, work and sex.

TERMINATION OF PREGNANCY

The definition of termination varies from one country to another. In the UK, it is defined as any pregnancy induced at < 24 weeks (UK) or < 500 g (WHO). Viability has been achieved lower than these parameters so that in reality the definitions are blurred.

Abortion is legal in the UK under the Abortion Act (1967):

- Category A   to save the mother's life
- Category B   to prevent grave permanent injury to the mother's physical or mental health
- Category C   if < 24 weeks, to avoid injury to the physical or mental health of the mother
- Category D   if < 24 weeks, to avoid injury to the physical or mental health of the existing child(ren)
- Category E   if the child is likely to be severely physically or mentally handicapped.

Counselling for 'social' (class C) terminations

Counselling is very important and should begin with an open invitation to talk. It is very useful to establish the views of the father of the baby, details of their relationship, and who else knows about the pregnancy. Often it can also be helpful to find out the woman's views about having children in the future, adoption and whether there are any future contraception plans.

The woman must be aware that there is a possibility, albeit rare, that infection after TOP may lead to tubal occlusion and secondary infertility. There is also a failure rate and either a clinical follow-up or pregnancy test 2–6 weeks after the termination is important. (Note: A pregnancy test may be positive for up to 4 weeks despite successful TOP.) It is important to either screen for and treat infections (including chlamydia), or treat all prophylactically (e.g. metronidazole 1 g PR (or 800 mg PO) and azithromycin 1 g PO).

Method

It is important to confirm that the woman is pregnant and to establish the gestation either clinically or by USS. Blood should be sent for grouping and antibodies, and anti-D given after termination to Rhesus-negative women. Options should be explained and the woman given the choice between suction termination (usually limited to < 12 weeks gestation) and medical termination.

URINARY INCONTINENCE

> Urinary incontinence is the involuntary loss of urine which is
> objectively demonstrated and which is a social problem. It can
> be broadly divided into 'genuine stress incontinence' (also
> referred to as 'urodynamic stress incontinence') caused by
> bladder neck weakness; and an 'unstable bladder' (or
> 'detrusor instability') caused by an over active detrusor
> muscle. A more detailed classification is shown in Figure 8.1.

History

- Is there stress incontinence (i.e. is there leakage when she laughs, coughs or sneezes)? This symptom suggests genuine stress incontinence, but is not pathognomonic of it.
- Is there urgency, urge incontinence, enuresis or continuous leakage? These suggest detrusor instability.
- How much does it affect lifestyle (important when considering surgery)?
- Is sanitary protection used (e.g. change of underwear, towels, mini-pads, large pads)?

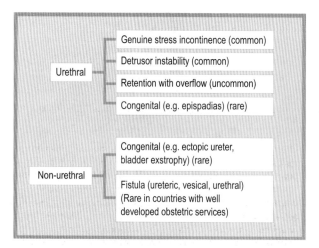

Fig. 8.1 Classification of urinary incontinence.

- Is fluid throughput thought to be high, average or low (normal ≈ 1500 ml/24 h)? If very high output, consider polydipsia and (rarely) diabetes insipidus.
- Nocturia (once or twice is normal); frequency, urgency, urge incontinence, enuresis and adverse effect of running water are features of detrusor instability.
- Dysuria suggests cystitis.
- Is there incontinence with intercourse? (leakage with penetration suggests stress incontinence and those with DI leak at orgasm).
- Haematuria can indicate malignancy (particularly in older women), but more commonly infection.
- Pushing or straining to void (± absent sensation) suggests outflow obstruction or detrusor hypocontractility or acontractility.
- Drug history, particularly diuretics and psychotropics.
- Has any treatment been tried (pelvic exercises, drugs, operations)?

Frequency–volume chart This provides a simple, objective 3-day method of assessing a patient's bladder function and habit. A record is kept of the time and volume of each urination. A normal woman passes about 1500 ml/24 h in 6–8 voids and the bladder capacity is usually (but not always) 300–500 ml. Any wide variation from this may indicate an abnormality (e.g. a total output of > 2000 ml is excessive unless there is a history of recurrent infection and an output < 1000 ml may predispose to infection). With DI, smaller volumes are passed more frequently day and night (e.g. 100–200 ml).

Clinical examination

- General examination. Is the patient obese?
- Pelvic examination:
  — Exclude a pelvic mass (may predispose to urgency).
  — Is there urinary leakage (confirms complaint)? Is there a cystocele (may predispose to GSI or obstruction with overflow)?
- Urinalysis for blood, sugar and protein. Send an MSU if positive.

Urodynamic investigations

These are indicated preoperatively, after failed surgery, for unusual symptoms, or in the presence of residual urine, recurrent infection or other abnormality (e.g. fistula). It may, for example, be important to differentiate GSI as a cause of stress incontinence from unstable detrusor contractions provoked by coughing. These investigations may not be universally available, however, and have a relatively low sensitivity and specificity. Some clinicians do not perform urodynamics on all preoperative patients with stress incontinence if there are no features in the history to suggest bladder instability.

Cystometry This is a method of assessing detrusor activity during a series of provocation tests such as with coughing, when voiding and on bladder filling. Intravesical pressure is composed of both transmitted abdominal pressure (e.g. coughing) and detrusor contraction pressure. Static cystometry therefore requires intravesical and intrarectal (= intra-abdominal) pressure lines and a urethral catheter to allow retrograde bladder filling. Detrusor activity may be observed by electronic subtraction or 'eyeballing' the record. After an initial independent flow rate to exclude obstruction, the residual volume is measured (normal < 50–100 ml). The bladder is then filled and the first desire to void noted (usually around 200 ml; earlier suggests DI). The total capacity is noted (usually > 400 ml; lower suggests DI). There should be no leakage with coughing (leakage in the absence of detrusor contraction indicates GSI), and no detrusor contractions during the filling phase until the patient is asked to void (contractions while the patient is trying to inhibit micturition suggests DI). Ambulatory cystometry is more time consuming, but may be more sensitive and specific.

Videocystometry (also known as video pressure/flow cystometry) This is used to observe bladder neck opening at rest or on coughing. It is also used to demonstrate leakage on provocation (e.g. coughing) and vesicoureteric reflux (e.g. patients with recurrent UTI).

Flow study This measures the rate of flow (normal > 15 ml/s). The flow rate is reduced in outflow obstruction (uncommon in women).

USS This measures residual urine volume (useful if there is possible retention, e.g. postoperatively, post-delivery).

Cystoscopy and IVU These are particularly appropriate with haematuria in the elderly, with recurrent UTI and to exclude chronic cystitis, stones and tumours.

Electromyography This may be indicated when neurological dysfunction is suspected.

GENUINE STRESS INCONTINENCE (GSI)

GSI is the involuntary loss of urine when intravesical pressure exceeds the maximum urethral closure pressure in the absence of detrusor activity. The more recent term to describe this is 'urodynamic stress incontinence' and requires, by definition, urodynamic testing (*www.rcog.org.uk*, Guideline 53). It is caused by either bladder neck hypermobility or intrinsic sphincter deficiency. Diagnosis is suggested by a history of leakage with coughing, laughing, sneezing or exercise, and may be supported by clinical examination and a frequency–volume chart. Cystometry is diagnostic, as the above stimuli may also provoke pathological detrusor contractions.

Conservative treatment for GSI

This is very effective in many patients and avoids the potentially serious complications of surgery. It should always be tried before considering surgery.

- Stop smoking (therefore less coughing) and lose weight.
- If mild, insertion of a tampon (e.g. before exercise) may be of help as a temporary measure.
- Pelvic floor exercises. The patient is advised to squeeze repeatedly (as if trying to stop the passage of flatus) for 2 minutes twice every day over a number of months. Alternatively 'cones', which are smooth graded tampon-like weights, can be inserted and held, the weight being increased as the muscle strength improves. These are preferable to midstream stops, which increase intravesical pressure and may lead to back-pressure on the kidneys.
- Electrical treatment to the vaginal muscles (e.g. interferential therapy). Pelvic floor exercises have been found to be more effective than electrical treatment or cones (BMJ 1999;318:487).
- There is conflicting evidence concerning the effect of oestrogens in the postmenopausal patient, but a topical preparation may be of benefit.

Surgical treatment for GSI

The choice of operation depends on the surgeon's preference, the patient's general health, the degree of prolapse and previous surgery. A choice may have to be made between cure rate and morbidity (e.g. retropubic bladder-neck elevation vs periurethral bulking agents). Surgery aims to elevate the bladder neck, but the mechanism by which this confers benefit remains controversial.

Surgery

- A 'clam' ileocystoplasty is a major undertaking and is for intractable DI only. A segment of ileum on a vascular pedicle is mobilized, opened longitudinally and sutured into the bladder vault to create a reservoir. The remaining ileum is re-anastomosed. Success rates of 50–90% have been reported, but the patient will be obliged to undertake regular intermittent self-catheterization and there are problems from mucus within the bladder. Long-term follow-up is required because of the risk of adenocarcinoma in the ileal segment.
- An ileal conduit with urostomy is an option for intractable cases.

FISTULAE

> Fistulae are often complex, multiple and are usually secondary to other causes. A pathological diagnosis is very important:
> - **malignancy (genital, GI, GU, metastatic or post-irradiation)**
> - **trauma (particularly surgery)**
> - **inflammation (IBD, diverticular disease, actinomycoses (e.g. with an IUCD), topical genital infections)**
> - **obstetric problems (necrosis and lacerations), generally only Third World.**

History

The history is usually of uncontrolled urinary and/or faecal leakage. Urinary leakage may be intermittent (e.g. only when the bladder is full) and, in the case of a uterovesical fistula, there may be cyclical haematuria. If there is an uncertain history of urinary leakage, it is useful to place a swab high in the vagina and fill the bladder with dye (e.g. methylene blue in normal saline) through a urethral catheter. The patient is asked to mobilize and the pad is inspected later for evidence of the dye. Otherwise EUA is the usual initial investigation, probing areas of granulation tissue gently to identify connections with bladder or bowel. Cystoscopy or sigmoidoscopy may confirm continuity of the probe outside the vagina. Imaging with colpography (catheter balloon in the vagina), fistulography, cystography, hysteroscopy, IVU and small bowel radiographs may also be helpful.

Management principles

- If the fistula occurs in the immediate postoperative period, consider arranging immediate closure.
- Closure of later postoperative fistulae should be delayed for 2–3 months to allow inflammation to settle.
- If there is malignancy, treat and consider diversion or exenteration.
- If there is IBD, treat medically before closure of the fistula.
- Do not close a urinary fistula if there is no residual sphincter, as this simply leads to incontinence from the urethra.
- Any urinary calculi must be removed before surgery.
- General health is important. Correct anaemia.

Surgical options

These should only be undertaken by someone with a subspecialist interest. Options include conservative management, laying open (e.g. for a low anal lesion in IBD), transvaginal closure in layers (e.g. for midvaginal fistulae), saucerization (closure with a purse-string suture if there is little extra tissue), or via the transabdominal route (using a transvesical or transperitoneal approach ± grafting). Ureteric fistulae may require construction using a Boari flap, or a loop of bowel, or re-anastomosis to the contralateral ureter.

GYNAECOLOGICAL ONCOLOGY

> All gynaecological cancers should be managed by a
> multidisciplinary team comprising a specialist gynaecologist,
> clinical/medical oncologist and palliative medicine specialist.
> Where possible, patients should be entered into trials.

BENIGN AND MALIGNANT DISEASE OF THE VULVA

Pruritus vulvae

This can affect any age group. Many disorders can cause itching and a
diagnosis should be possible in most cases, sometimes with a need for
biopsy. If the diagnosis is uncertain, consider referral to a specialist
vulval clinic, where the combined input of a dermatologist and a
gynaecologist are available. Causes:

- Infection (candida, diabetes mellitus/HIV, pediculosis, scabies,
  threadworms, trichomonas, bacterial vaginosis, herpes simplex,
  UTI).
- Dermatological conditions (contact and seborrhoeic
  dermatitis/eczema, lichen sclerosis, lichen simplex, lichen planus,
  squamous cell hyperplasia, symptomatic dermatographism).
- Neoplasia (squamous cell carcinoma – in young women the
  background is likely to be VIN and in the elderly, lichen sclerosis;
  melanoma, basal cell carcinoma and Bartholin's gland carcinoma).
- Other causes (oestrogen withdrawal; gastrointestinal disease;
  urinary incontinence; pregnancy; any cause of systemic pruritus,
  e.g. drugs, renal or hepatic impairment, lymphoma, psychological).
- Idiopathic – uncommon and can only be made when all causes
  excluded.

Management should be to treat any underlying cause first. Vulval skin
is sensitive therefore avoid soaps and detergents, tight-fitting clothing,
spermicidally lubricated and/or latex condoms. Symptomatic relief can
be obtained in the form of emollients and soap substitutes (e.g.
Dermol 600, Oilatum), corticosteroids (betamethasone 0.1% BD to
QID for 2–3 weeks then hydrocortisone 1% BD to OD or less as
maintenance). Written patient information leaflets are useful.

VULVODYNIA (LANCET 2004:363:1058)

This is chronic vulval discomfort, especially that characterized by the
complaint of burning, stinging, irritation or rawness. It is used to

describe the presence of symptoms for over 3 months without any
visible lesion. Cumulative lifetime incidence may be around 15%.
There are two conditions that are part of the vulvodynia spectrum:
vulval vestibulitis and dysaesthetic vulvodynia. Vulval vestibulitis is
characterized by severe pain on vestibular touch or attempted vaginal
entry, tenderness to pressure localized within the vulval vestibule, and
physical findings of erythema limited to the vulval vestibule. It tends
to occur in white premenopausal women who are sexually active.
Dysaesthetic vulvodynia describes unprovoked vulval burning not
limited to the vestibule and with no demonstrable abnormalities. It
occurs more frequently in older women and the pain can extend
beyond the vulva to the thigh or anus. Although vulvodynia is
associated with depressive symptoms there is little evidence for a link
to physical or sexual abuse. Useful interventions include tricyclic
antidepressants, gabapentin, acupuncture, pelvic floor exercises with
biofeedback, 5% lidocaine (lignocaine) cream and interferon. The
Vulval Pain Society is a self-help group for patients with vulvodynia
(www.vul-pain.dircon.co.uk).

Ulcers

These may be:

- aphthous (yellow base)
- herpetic (exquisitely painful multiple ulceration, p. 255)
- syphilitic (indurated and painless, p. 256)
- related to Crohn's disease (like knife cuts in the skin)
- a feature of Behçet's disease (chronic painful condition with
  aphthous, genital and ocular ulceration. Treatment: OCP or topical
  steroids)
- neoplastic
- associated with lichen planus or Stevens–Johnson syndrome
- tropical (lymphogranuloma venereum, chancroid, granuloma
  inguinale).

ISSVD classification for benign vulval diseases

Lichen sclerosis This can present at any age but most commonly in
older age groups, and occasionally in childhood (can be mistaken for
sexual abuse). It usually presents with itch. There is an association
with autoimmune disorders in < 10% (alopecia areata and vitiligo are
the most common but also PA, thyroid disease, IDDM, SLE, primary
biliary cirrhosis or bullous pemphigoid). The skin appears white and
thin but may be thickened and keratotic if there is co-existing
squamous cell hyperplasia. There may be clitoral or labial adhesions.
Diagnosis is best by biopsy – which may be done under local

anaesthetic. It may co-exist with VIN and 4–5% will subsequently develop carcinoma of the vulva so that long-term follow up is required. Treatment is only necessary if there are significant symptoms, e.g. clobetasol 0.05% BD (Dermovate) for 2–3 months reducing gradually to hydrocortisone 1% sparingly as required. Vulvectomy has no role as there is a high rate of recurrence.

Squamous cell hyperplasia This frequently presents in premenopausal women with severe pruritus. Diagnosis is by biopsy and treatment is as for lichen sclerosis.

Other dermatoses

- *Contact dermatosis*. This may be caused by detergents, perfume, condom lubricants, chlorine from swimming pools, etc. There may be secondary infection. Exclude the irritant and treat as for 'pruritus vulvae'.
- *Psoriasis*. The vulva is an unusual site for this but if it is present, moderately potent steroids are better than coal tar.
- *Intertrigo*. Along with candida, this responds to antifungal preparations.
- *Lichen planus*. This appears as purple white papules with a shiny surface and keratinized area and may respond to potent steroids +/– azathioprine or PUVA. It is usually idiopathic, but can be drug related, and tends to resolve within 2 years. Avoid surgery.

VARIETIES OF INTRAEPITHELIAL NEOPLASIA (NOTE: NEOPLASTIC CELLS ARE CONFINED TO THE EPITHELIUM)

Squamous vulval intraepithelial neoplasia (VIN) 'VIN' is preferred to previous eponymous terms. Depending on severity it can be classified as 1, 2, or 3, although there is a lack of consensus between pathologists and clinicians regarding VIN terminology (some prefer to use 'high grade' and 'low grade'). Unlike CIN there is less evidence for a progressive process. HPV and smoking are likely to be aetiological factors. Many women are asymptomatic although pruritus is the most common presenting symptom with pain an occasional feature. Lesions may be papular and rough surfaced, resembling warts, or macular with indistinct borders. White lesions represent hyperkeratosis and pigmentation is common. The lesions tend to be multifocal in women under 40 and unifocal in the postmenopausal age group. Diagnosis is made by biopsy. Treatment is controversial as the natural history is unknown. Regression has been known but progression to high-grade VIN or invasion may occur in approximately 6% of cases and up to 15% of those with VIN 3 may have superficial invasion. The main treatment is wide local excision, but laser ablation (Nd-YAG or CO_2) can also be used. Newer treatment includes the use of topical imiquimod (unlicensed), but the use of topical 5-fluorouracil has not been shown to be beneficial.

Non-squamous VIN (Paget's disease) This is uncommon. There is a poorly demarcated, often multifocal eczematoid lesion associated in 25% with adenocarcinoma either in the pelvis or at a distant site. Treatment is by wide local excision.

Melanoma in-situ This is rare.

VULVAL CARCINOMA

> **Vulval carcinoma is a rare tumour with only 1000 new cases in the UK every year. The overall 5-year survival rate is < 50%. It most commonly presents in the elderly with 80% occurring in the over 65-year age group. Commonly there is pruritus vulvae (70%), ulcer or mass (57%) or bleeding (25%). The majority of lesions occur on the labia majora (50%) (especially anteriorly), the labia minora accounting for 15–20% and the rest on the clitoris, posterior fourchette, and perineum. Spread is by embolization to the locoregional lymphatics, the inguinofemoral lymph nodes and prognosis is inversely related to extent of spread. Haematogenous spread is unusual. Diagnosis is with EUA and excision biopsy, although outpatient biopsy may be appropriate (ultrasound guided FNA of groin nodes has been reported as having a specificity and sensitivity approaching 100%). MRI, ultrasound and lymphoscintigraphy have increasing potential to diagnose lymph node involvement. It is essential to examine the cervix and perform a smear to exclude co-existing CIN or cervical carcinoma.**

Histology of vulval malignancy

- Approximately 85% are squamous cell carcinoma (SCC).
- Approximately 5% are malignant melanomas.
- Basal cell carcinoma and verrucous carcinoma are rare.
- Adenocarcinoma arising from Bartholin's or paraurethral glands is also rare.

Surgical treatment

See Table 9.1 for the staging of vulval carcinoma.

Two-thirds of cases are early stage which carry a 5-year survival rate of 80–90%. Survival with nodal disease diminishes to 40%. Factors predictive of nodal disease are: clinically suspicious groin nodes, grade of tumour (more likely if poorly differentiated), age of patient (more likely if older) and presence of lymphatic or vascular space invasion. Depth of stromal invasion is particularly related to groin node involvement:

- < 1 mm   No positive groin nodes
- < 3 mm   12% positive groin nodes
- < 5 mm   16% positive groin nodes.

Management of vulval carcinoma is showing a trend to more conservative surgery aiming to preserve organ function without affecting chance of cure. Treatment is wide local excision for IA tumours (i.e. excision which includes a 10 mm margin of normal tissue laterally and deep to the tumour). For lateralized stage IB/II disease (i.e. a lesion where the surgical excision line will not include a midline structure [e.g. clitoris, anus, urethra or vagina] by a minimum margin of 10 mm) treatment is wide local excision + ipsilateral groin node dissection. Contralateral groin node exploration is only carried out if the ipsilateral groin nodes are positive (if the ipsilateral groin nodes are negative the risk of contralateral groin node involvement is < 1%). If the disease involves a midline structure, wide local excision and bilateral groin node dissection is appropriate.

TABLE 9.1 Staging of vulval carcinoma (FIGO 1995)

Stage	Criteria
IA	Tumour less than 2.0 cm in dimension and less than 1 mm of stromal invasion. No nodal metastasis
IB	Tumour less than 2.0 cm in dimension but with more than 1 mm of stromal invasion. No nodal metastasis
II	Tumour of more than 2.0 cm dimension confined to vulva or perineum with no nodal metastasis
III	Tumour of any size with (i) adjacent spread to the lower urethra and/or vagina or anus, and/or (ii) unilateral regional lymph node metastasis
IVA	Tumour invades any of the following: upper urethra, bladder mucosa, rectal mucosa, pelvic bone +/– bilateral groin nodes
IVB	Any distant metastases including pelvic nodes

Groin lymphadenectomy carries significant morbidity. The wounds should be drained for at least 7–10 days, otherwise lymph collection or lymphocyst formation and wound breakdown can occur. Lower limb lymphoedema can cause serious long-term morbidity. Less invasive methods of diagnosing groin involvement would reduce the need for groin surgery and its sequelae. The introduction of sentinel lymph node sampling using preoperative lymphoscintigraphy with radioactive technetium is a promising technique for staging without the need for invasive surgery. For larger lesions, radical wide local excision may be appropriate but the risk of recurrence is high if the resection margin is < 8 mm. Otherwise radical vulval resection is the operation of choice. Involvement of a plastic surgeon may be necessary for satisfactory wound closure.

For locally advanced disease the distal third of the urethra can be excised without compromising continence. Anorectal involvement requires proctectomy and stoma formation as well as radical vulvectomy and bilateral groin node dissection. Such radical surgery has a mortality of nearly 10% with considerable psychological morbidity. Clinical nurse specialists can aid recovery enormously. Most patients will require adjuvant radiotherapy for stage III and above disease. This usually involves external beam radiotherapy but electron or brachytherapy may be required where the primary tumour is inoperable. Chemotherapy is generally reserved for inoperable local disease, recurrent or metastatic disease.

OTHER TUMOURS

Malignant melanoma This is the second most common malignancy of the vulva. Wide local excision is the primary treatment. Prognosis is principally dependent on the depth of invasion (Breslow thickness) – if there is < 0.76 mm then nodal metastasis is rare, and if there is > 2 mm the prognosis worsens.

Bartholin's gland carcinoma A mass in the Bartholin's gland of a post-menopausal patient should be considered malignant until proven otherwise. Average age of presentation is 60 years. Surgical management is as for squamous cell carcinoma with radiotherapy for positive resection margins or metastatic disease.

Basal cell carcinoma These constitute 2–4% of vulval cancers. Local excision is usually curative.

Verrucous carcinoma This appears like a giant wart. It is a variant of squamous cell carcinoma, is slow-growing, and tends to local invasion. Treatment is wide local excision but without nodal dissection. Radiotherapy can cause a more aggressive form to occur and recurrences are therefore treated with re-excision.

Rare tumours These include Merkel-cell carcinoma, sarcoma, leiomyosarcoma, malignant fibrous histiocytoma, dermatofibrosarcoma protuberans, rhabdomyosarcoma, epithelioid sarcoma, Kaposi's sarcoma, vulval lymphoma and metastatic disease. Most are highly aggressive tumours with distant metastases at presentation.

CERVICAL SMEARS

Cervical smears are used to detect dyskaryosis (changes in individual cells with hyperchromasia, irregular nuclei and multinucleation) in cells of the cervical epithelium. The aim of the smear programme is to screen for precancerous changes in the cervical epithelium (cervical intraepithelial neoplasia or CIN) which can be treated, thereby reducing the incidence of cervical cancer. Dyskaryosis is classified as mild, moderate and severe and suggests referral for colposcopy where biopsy or treatment can take place. Cervical screening is offered to all women between the ages of 25 to 64 years (20–60 years in Scotland) at least every 5 years but more usually every 3 years. Annual smears increase overall cost with little increase in detection rate. There is some evidence to suggest that screening may be discontinued on reaching the age of 50 with a normal smear history, as the risk of malignancy is so low in this group. The introduction of liquid-based cytology (where smears are placed in a liquid medium rather than smeared on a glass slide) has significantly lowered the number of unsatisfactory smears and improved both sensitivity and specificity.

Cervical smears must not be offered to women under 20 years as the incidence of cervical cancer in this group is low and the prevalence of transient HPV infection after coitarche high. Much low-grade disease would regress and they are at risk of over-treatment if screening is commenced. Only those attending colposcopy or with HIV or other causes of immunosuppression should have annual or more frequent smears.

Screening is based on the assumption that CIN is a progressive disorder from CIN 1 to CIN 3 and invasive carcinoma. The risk of CIN 3 progressing to invasive disease is uncertain, but estimates range from 14% to 70%. With CIN 1 30–60% regress and 10–30% may progress to CIN 3. Longitudinal studies have shown that CIN 3 may progress to invasive carcinoma in 30–70% of cases over a period of 10–12 years. Cervical smears are also used for surveillance following colposcopy and vault smears may be used for follow-up after treatment for cervical cancer. An example of management of the abnormal smear is shown in Table 9.2.

Notes

- Glandular neoplasia may be detected on cervical smears (CGIN) and should be seen urgently as 40% will have invasive disease. Colposcopy is poor at detecting CGIN or invasive adenocarcinoma; the majority are diagnosed after large loop excision. A glandular abnormality on a smear should prompt investigation of the uterus and ovaries (TVUS + hysteroscopy or endometrial biopsy). Those with inadequate smears are also at increased risk of pre-invasive

TABLE 9.2 Cervical cytology, associated pathology and subsequent management			
Smear	Risk of having CIN II or III on biopsy	Management	If next smear(s) negative then
Normal	0.1%	Repeat in 3 years if no previous abnormality	Routine recall
Inflammatory	< 6%	Repeat in 3 years if no previous abnormality	Routine recall
Borderline	20–37%	Repeat in 6 months	Repeat in 1 year, then 2 years then routine recall Colposcopy if 3 borderline
Mild dyskaryosis	30–50% (note that 30% have CIN I, 30–60% regress and 10% may progress to CIN III)	Repeat in 3 months	Repeat in 1 year, then 2 years then routine recall Colposcopy if 2 mild dyskaryosis
Moderate dyskaryosis	50–70%	Colposcopy	Repeat at follow-up
Severe dyskaryosis	80–90%	Colposcopy	Repeat at follow-up
Invasion suspected	50% have invasion	Urgent colposcopy	

disease (17–40%) and should be referred to colposcopy if three consecutive smears are reported as inadequate or unsatisfactory.

- Koilocytosis suggest papilloma virus infection. A useful tool in the future may be testing for oncogenic forms of HPV (principally 16 and 18) which may help to distinguish which low grade forms of CIN are likely to progress.
- Other infections such as candida, trichomonas, gardnarella, chlamydia and gonococcus can be diagnosed from cervical smears using LBC.

COLPOSCOPY

> **The transformation zone (TZ) is a circumferential region of tissue between the vaginal (squamous) and the endocervical (columnar) epithelium. The columnar epithelium undergoes metaplasia to squamous epithelium in response to the low pH of the vagina. It is this area that has to be inspected at colposcopy.**

Many patients have a high degree of anxiety (e.g. fear of cancer, intimate examination) on attending colposcopy which can be reduced by sending written information out prior to the appointment.

Other indications for referral include: abnormal or suspicious cervix, postcoital bleeding (young women may be referred to GUM as infection is a more likely cause of PCB). Note: contact bleeding at the time of smear taking is in itself not an indication for referral.

History, examination and investigation

Clinicians undertaking colposcopy treatment should be suitably trained and registered with the BSCCP (*www.bsccp.org.uk*). Take a history (preferably using a standard proforma, which allows easy auditing, and concentrates on symptoms relevant to cervical disease). Insert a speculum looking for vulval disease, condylomata and invasive cervical disease – a cauliflower appearance with ulceration or atypical vessels.

Apply 3–5% acetic acid. This coagulates protein and stains abnormal cells (which have a more rapid turnover and therefore more protein) white:

- Columnar epithelium blanches white briefly and has a villous surface.

- Squamous metaplasia appears glassy white and can be hard to differentiate from CIN.
- HPV infection can appear as small lesions with looped capillaries +/– satellite lesions.
- CIN; dense white with more high grade CIN showing abnormal vessels alone or in a mosaic pattern or 'punctuation' when the vessels are seen end on.

The application of Lugol's iodine (Schiller's test) stains glycogen in normal cells mahogany brown. Non-staining areas are termed Schiller's negative.

Management

Adequate visualization of the TZ is essential before colposcopy can be deemed to be satisfactory. If any abnormality is seen, biopsy is required. Treatment and biopsy in the form of large loop excision (LLETZ) may be offered at the first visit – 'see and treat' policy. The alternative is to take a smaller biopsy and review later to decide if LLETZ is required. To perform LLETZ infiltrate the paracervical tissue with Citanest and Octapressin, excise to a depth of at least 7 mm (preferably in one sample), and administer diathermy to the base. Advise the patient to expect watery, blood-stained discharge for up to 3 weeks, and to avoid tampon use and intercourse while this is present; pain or heavier bleeding several days post-operatively suggests infection and may merit antibiotics.

CIN 1 may be kept under review but if it continues for > 24 months suggest LLETZ.

Notes

- The squamocolumnar junction is marked by the lower limit of the columnar epithelium, not the upper limit of squamous epithelium.
- If the TZ is not seen, a deep LLETZ is appropriate.
- Destructive methods of treatment (cold coagulation, laser) must not be performed unless a biopsy has been taken previously, and never for suspected invasive disease or cervical glandular intraepithelial neoplasia.
- If CGIN is suspected, biopsy is mandatory as colposcopy is less reliable. If cervical glandular intraepithelial neoplasia is confirmed excise with LLETZ or a cold knife (cone biopsy). Consider hysterectomy if the family is complete, if there are positive margins after excisional procedure, or if there is failure to achieve cytological follow-up, e.g. due to cervical stenosis.
- In a previously treated cervix, excision is preferable to ablation.

- Hysterectomy is appropriate treatment for a patient with high-grade disease who has completed her family, or has co-existing menstrual dysfunction and who wishes curative treatment. Although risk of vaginal intraepithelial neoplasia (VaIN) is small (1%), follow-up smears are recommended at 6 and 18 months. If negative, no further smears are indicated.
- If cervical disease is extensive, a good cuff of vagina should be taken to avoid VaIN in the 'dog ears' at the vault. Around 30% of VaIN progresses to invasive disease.

CERVICAL CANCER

The cervical screening programme has significantly reduced the incidence of this disease. Estimates are that 1 in 80 of the 8 million British women born between 1951 and 1970 will be saved from premature death by the cervical screening programme at a cost per life saved of about £36 000 (Lancet 2004; 364: 249). Most cases are now picked up at an earlier stage as a result.

Clinical presentation is with intermenstrual or postcoital bleeding (*any* patient with these symptoms *must* have a speculum examination) or, much more rarely, with loin pain and renal failure in advanced disease. Spread is to the internal and external iliac, obturator and common iliac nodes then to para-aortic nodes. Tumour can also invade locally to involve bladder, ureters, rectum and bone. Blood-borne metastases to liver, lungs and bone can occur.

Histology

- Almost 90% are squamous cell. Oncogenic HPV (most commonly types 16 and 18) is a major cause. Other associated factors are linked to acquisition of this: age at first intercourse, number of partners, smoking, OCP use, chlamydia infection and immunocompromise.
- About 10% are adenocarcinoma.
- There are other rare possibilities. Adenosquamous has a worse prognosis than squamous cell. Malignant melanoma, sarcoma, lymphoma and small cell carcinoma can all occur.

Staging

This is *clinical*, based on EUA, speculum and rectovaginal examination (to assess parametrial involvement), cystoscopy, curettage and biopsy +/– IVU. Although not part of the staging process, CT or MRI are increasingly used to assess the size of the tumour and nodal metastases. If nodes are suspicious and the cervical lesion is < 4 cm in diameter, chemo/radiotherapy may be more appropriate treatments than surgery. See Table 9.3.

Notes

- Prognosis is strongly linked to stage. See Table 9.3.
- It is uncertain whether lymphovascular space invasion increases risk of nodal metastasis in Stage IA disease.
- If pelvic nodes are positive, up to 60% have positive para-aortic nodes.
- Lymph node metastasis is associated with poorer prognosis.
- Several studies have shown a benefit of combined chemo- (cisplatin) and radiotherapy.

Management

Treatment should be tailored to the individual and where possible the individual should be enrolled into a randomized controlled trial. For small tumours, radiotherapy is as effective as surgery, but surgery causes less long-term morbidity. Ovaries should be conserved in young women.

Radical (Wertheim's) hysterectomy and bilateral pelvic lymphadenectomy This carries an operative mortality < 1% with a subsequent risk of infection, VTE, haemorrhage, vesicovaginal and uretovaginal fistulae. Medium-term complications include voiding difficulties (overcome by suprapubic catheterization and bladder 'retraining'), recurrent UTI and stress incontinence. There is a current trend to move towards laparoscopic surgery as nodal dissection may be easier and the inpatient stay is shorter with quicker return to normal functioning. Operative time however may be increased.

Radiotherapy Generally, this is radical pelvic radiotherapy with external beam X-ray treatment (teletherapy) to the pelvis. Ensure there are no distant metastases before commencing treatment. Treatment is given in 20 fractions over 4 weeks. It may also be given as parallel opposed fields or anterior and posterior fields. This is usually followed by an intracavitary treatment (brachytherapy) where a vaginal delivery system is inserted under anaesthesia and the radiation delivered by a Selectron machine taking 12–18 hours. The patient is awake during treatment and discomfort may be relieved by a caudal block or sedation. Some patients will require a second insertion 2–3 weeks after the first. Acute diarrhoea can be treated with low residue diet and Imodium or codeine.

TABLE 9.3 FIGO staging of cervical cancer

Stage	Invasion	Pelvic nodes	Para-aortic nodes	Prognosis 5-year survival	Treatment
IA1	Depth of invasion < 3 mm and width < 7 mm	< 1%	0%	Nearly 100%	Conization if the patient wishes fertility; if not, simple hysterectomy
	With lymphovascular space invasion				Simple hysterectomy +/– lymphadenectomy
IA2	Depth of invasion between 3–5 mm and width < 7 mm	6.5%	0%	Nearly 100%	Radical hysterectomy and pelvic lymphadenectomy
IB1	Tumour confined to cervix and diameter < 4 cm	15%		70–85%	Radical hysterectomy and pelvic lymphadenectomy plus chemoradiotherapy for poor prognostic factors
IB2	Tumour confined to cervix and diameter > 4 cm	15%	5%	70–85%	Radiotherapy + chemotherapy
IIA	Upper 2/3 vagina	25%	15%	62%	Radiotherapy + chemotherapy

(Continued)

TABLE 9.3 FIGO staging of cervical cancer (Continued)

Stage	Invasion	Pelvic nodes	Para-aortic nodes	Prognosis 5-year survival	Treatment
IIB	Upper 2/3 vagina + parametrial disease			50–70%	Radiotherapy + chemotherapy
IIIA	Lower 1/3 vagina	35%	25%	30–50%	
IIIB	Pelvic side wall +/– hydronephrosis			30–50%	
IVA	Bladder, rectum	50%	40%	5–15%	
IVB	Beyond pelvis			5–15%	

Long-term side-effects of radiotherapy occur in 5–10% and include diarrhoea, radiation cystitis, radiation proctitis (rectal bleeding) and vaginal stenosis.

Recurrence

- *After surgery*: give radiotherapy +/– chemotherapy.
- *After radiotherapy*: if recurrence is small and central with no evidence of nodal spread, pelvic exenteration should be considered, with urinary and bowel diversion if required, and pelvic floor reconstruction. Operative mortality is 10–20% and there is major morbidity. Five-year survival is 30%.

ENDOMETRIAL CANCER

This is the commonest gynaecological malignancy with over 4500 new cases annually in the UK. More than 80% occur in postmenopausal women. Risk factors include low parity, late menopause, obesity, PCOS, unopposed oestrogen preparations, tamoxifen, diabetes mellitus and hypertension. Breast-feeding, smoking and exercise are protective. Those with HNPCC (see Epithelial ovarian cancer, p. 329) are at higher risk. Presentation is usually with abnormal bleeding. A postmenopausal woman with a pyometrium should be considered to have carcinoma until proven otherwise.

Investigation of postmenopausal bleeding

There is good evidence for the use of transvaginal ultrasound (TVS) as the initial investigation. This also allows assessment of the adnexae. Good views of the endometrium are necessary and the thickness is measured in millimetres. If it is < 4 mm the risk of malignancy is so low that further investigation may not be necessary. If it is > 4 mm, biopsy either with aspiration (e.g. Pipelle) or hysteroscopy/D&C is necessary. With HRT use, this cut-off can be raised to 5 mm (*www.sign.ac.uk,* guideline 61). Women on tamoxifen should proceed directly to hysteroscopy/D&C.

Histology

- Adenocarcinoma is by far the most common and can be endometrioid (75–80%), uterine papillary serous (<10%), clear cell (4%), mucinous (1%), ciliated, secretory, papillary or

villoglandular, adenocarcinoma with squamous metaplasia, adenoacanthoma or adenosquamous.
- Squamous.
- Mixed.
- Undifferentiated.
- Other uterine malignancies are rare and include: mixed mesodermal tumour (carcinosarcoma), leiomyosarcoma, endometrial stromal sarcoma. These are more aggressive tumours and prognosis is often poor.

Treatment

Staging is surgical (Table 9.4). At laparotomy perform peritoneal washings (although management of early stage disease with positive cytology is uncertain) and examine for omental, para-aortic and hepatic spread. A TAH and BSO should be carried out but lymphadenectomy is controversial. The MRC 'ASTEC' trial is nearing completion and may report in the near future.

Prognosis is dependent not only on the stage but the patient's age, histological grade (G1 better that 3) and cell ploidy (euploidy better).

Postoperative treatment

In most cases of stage I disease, surgery is curative but the recurrence rate for high risk cases can approach 50%. Radiotherapy for stage I

Stage	Definition	Pelvic nodes	5-year survival
TABLE 9.4 FIGO staging of endometrial carcinoma			
IA IB IC	Tumour limited to the endometrium Growth that has invaded < 50% of myometrial thickness Growth that has invaded > 50% of myometrial thickness	< 20%	70%
IIA IIB	Endocervical glandular involvement only Cervical stromal involved	20%	56%
IIIA IIIB IIIC	Invades serosal surface of uterus, +/– adnexa, +/– positive washings Vaginal metastases Metastases to pelvic or para-aortic nodes	35%	30%
IVA IVB	Tumour invasion of bladder and/or bowel Distant metastases including intra-abdominal and/or inguinal lymph nodes	50%	20%

disease has not been shown to improve survival but does reduce local recurrence albeit with increased morbidity. Radiotherapy with stage I disease is generally reserved for those with poor prognostic indicators (high grade, adenosquamous, clear cell or papillary serous tumours or deep myometrial invasion). For more advanced disease, chemotherapy is also indicated (a platinum-based regimen with doxorubicin and cyclophosphamide). Progesterone therapy does not convey any survival advantage but this may depend on tumour receptor status.

Recurrent disease

This is associated with poor prognosis. With central isolated recurrence, exenteration may achieve cure. Treatment will depend on previous management, as previous radiotherapy may make surgery or secondary radiotherapy futile. Most relapses occur within 2 years. Recurrence is commonest in lungs, bone, vagina, liver, inguinal and supraclavicular lymph nodes.

Up to 75% may respond to progesterone therapy (medroxyprogesterone acetate 30–100 mg TID) depending on receptor status. Those positive for the oestrogen receptor may respond to tamoxifen (20 mg daily). Negative receptor status appears to improve response rates to chemotherapy. These patients are suitable for entry into trials.

Follow-up

There are no adequate prospective studies for guidance and follow-up will depend on clinician preference and the individual patient's case. Several retrospective studies have failed to show any survival advantage of intensive surveillance but do show increased costs. Vault smears do not appear to improve detection of recurrence. An example of a follow-up regimen might be 3 monthly for the first year then 6 monthly for 2 years and yearly until 10 years.

FALLOPIAN TUBE TUMOURS

These are very rare. Peak incidence is at 60–64 years of age. Most present with serosanguinous discharge or bleeding and/or pelvic pain. These tumours can be considered a possibility in women with persisting postmenopausal bleeding and normal curettage. TVS may help with diagnosis – a sausage shaped mass with projections into a fluid-filled lumen is evident. More than 90% are papillary adenocarcinomas. FIGO staging is analogous to ovarian cancer staging, and treatment is also as for ovarian cancer with laparotomy, TAH/BSO omentectomy and cytoreduction. Adjuvant therapy in the form of chemotherapy is required for advanced disease. Overall 5-year survival for stages I and II is 50% and for stages III and IV it is 14%.

EPITHELIAL OVARIAN CANCER

More common in the postmenopausal age group, half of women developing the disease are over 65 years. Risk factors include: nulliparity, positive family history of breast or ovarian cancer (although > 90% are spontaneous). Risk of ovarian cancer appears to be linked to the number of ovulatory cycles experienced in a lifetime (i.e. increases with early menarche, late menopause, having first child after age 30, possibly use of ovulation induction in infertility treatment; COCP and breast-feeding protect), or genetic predisposition (see below). Presentation is often at a late stage – usually with abdominal pain and/or swelling; it can also present with vague abdominal symptoms, urinary frequency, weight loss, abnormal vaginal bleeding, leg/groin pain (with DVT) – hence the poor overall survival. Despite advances in chemotherapy, survival has not improved and < 30% are alive at 5 years. The pattern of disease is usually one of remission following surgery and chemotherapy, with relapse and development of tumour resistance to chemotherapeutic drugs some months or years later.

Pathology of ovarian tumours
These can be subdivided into:

- epithelial – (over 90% of ovarian tumours)
- germ cell
- sex cord/stromal
- miscellaneous and metastatic.

The last three are discussed in the next section. Epithelial tumours can be further subdivided:

Serous

- cystadenoma, papillary cystadenoma, or cystadenofibroma
- adenocarcinoma.

Mucinous

- Cystadenoma – multilocular. Rupture may lead to pseudomyxoma peritonei – a condition where there is widespread mucin within the peritoneal cavity. This can also arise from the gastrointestinal tract therefore the appendix should be inspected/removed.

TABLE 9.5 FIGO staging of ovarian cancer

Stage	Definition	5 year survival
IA	One ovary	85% overall,
IB	Both ovaries	and 95% for
IC	IA or IB with ruptured capsule, tumour on the surface of the capsule, positive peritoneal washings or malignant ascites	stage IA
IIA	Extension to uterus and tubes	
IIB	Extension to other pelvis tissues, e.g. pelvic nodes, pouch of Douglas	30–57%
IIC	IIA or IIB with ruptured capsule, positive peritoneal washings or malignant ascites	
IIIA	Pelvic tumour with microscopic peritoneal spread	
IIIB	Pelvic tumour with peritoneal spread < 2 cm	10–28%
IIIC	Abdominal implants > 2 cm +/– positive retroperitoneal or inguinal nodes	
IV	Liver parenchymal disease. Distant metastases. If pleural effusion, must have malignant cells	< 10%

quality of life, improve response to chemotherapy, prolong remission and increase median survival. Some surgeons would consider pelvic and para-aortic node sampling to ensure accurate staging in apparent Stage I disease.

Postoperative chemotherapy is usually given within 8 weeks of surgery. If optimal surgery has been performed for low-grade stage IA or IIA disease, chemotherapy may be deferred. However two RCTs have shown improved survival and reduced risk of relapse with carboplatin in early disease (www.sign.ac.uk, guideline 75). For more advanced disease, first-line chemotherapy should include a platinum-based drug either as a single agent or in combination with a taxane. Carboplatin and cisplatin have equivalent efficacies but cisplatin causes greater toxicity and carboplatin is easier to give as an outpatient. The combination of paclitaxel and carboplatin appears to have a slight survival benefit but causes more toxicity (especially neurotoxicity, allergic reaction and alopecia) than carboplatin alone. Therefore single agent carboplatin is more suitable for those unable to tolerate taxanes. Cyclophosphamide is no longer in use as a first line agent and there is no role for anthracyclines outside random controlled trials.

NON-EPITHELIAL OVARIAN CANCER

These account for ≈10% of ovarian malignancies. They tend to occur in women of reproductive age. Preoperative investigations should include αFP, hCG, lactate dehydrogenase (LDH), inhibin and oestradiol. CT is important to assess nodal enlargement if lymphadenectomy is not performed. Staging is as for epithelial ovarian cancer. Surgery is usually more conservative – unilateral salpingo-oophorectomy.

Germ cell tumours

These are uncommon but aggressive and are usually found in young women or adolescents – the peak incidence is in the early twenties. The most common is dysgerminoma: If they are diagnosed early they are potentially curable. Chemotherapy has improved prognosis.

- *Dysgerminoma* (a completely undifferentiated tumour). Female equivalent of seminoma. Accounts for 50% of malignant germ cell tumours and usually presents in the < 30-year-old age group. Approximately 10–15% have bilateral disease. They are very radio- and chemosensitive, but are treated with chemotherapy (BEP – bleomycin, etoposide and cisplatin) to preserve ovarian function. Good prognosis with overall survival of 90%.
- *Yolk sac tumour (= endodermal sinus tumour)*. These occur in the 14–20-year-old age group and secrete αFP. They are usually unilateral and chemosensitive. Rapidly growing, they present with abdominal pain and a pelvic mass. A histological feature is the Schiller–Duval body. Most recurrences are in the first year and it carries high mortality.
- *Malignant teratoma*. Most common in the first 2 decades of life. It is nearly always unilateral and often contains neural tissue. May secrete thyroid hormones (struma ovarii) and serotonin (carcinoid). Treatment involves surgery then chemotherapy.
- *Mature cystic teratoma (dermoid)*. Ninety percent occur in women of reproductive age. Ten to fifteen percent are bilateral. It is usually unilocular with a focal hillock, squamous epithelium and skin appendages. One percent have a focus of malignant change and these carry a poor prognosis.
- *Ovarian choriocarcinoma*. These secrete hCG and may present with precocious pseudopuberty. They have a poor prognosis and do not respond well to chemotherapy (unlike the GTD equivalent, p. 241).
- *Embryonal cancer* is rare. It may secrete αFP.
- *Mixed germ cell tumours* account for 8%, with dysgerminoma being the most common constituent.

- *Polyembryomas* are highly malignant and not sensitive to radiotherapy or chemotherapy.

Sex cord-stromal tumours

The majority are granulosa cell tumours and they can occur at any age. Surgery is treatment of choice and can be conservative especially in younger patient.

- Granulosa cell tumour:
  — Adult: The mean age is 52 years. Most produce oestradiol which can cause endometrial hyperplasia or even carcinoma. Some are androgenic. Inhibin is a tumour marker. Most are stage I and unilateral. It can occur years after apparent cure therefore it requires long-term follow-up. Prognosis is often good – 5-year survival is 80% (poor prognosis with advanced stage and recurrence).
  — Juvenile: Unilateral and large. Five per cent are malignant and usually aggressive. It can present with precocious puberty. It is treated with chemotherapy.
- Sertoli stromal cell tumours: These tumours contain Sertoli cells, Leydig cells or both, and can occur at any age. They may secrete oestrogen, androgens (androblastoma or arrhenoblastoma) and low level αFP. They most commonly present with menstrual disturbance in premenopausal women. Treatment is usually surgery then chemotherapy.
- Other: Includes gynandroblastoma, lipid cell tumour and unclassified(really unclassifiable).

Metastatic tumour In ovaries

About 10% are secondary tumours, most commonly from endometrium, then stomach, colon, breast, lung and pancreas. Krukenberg tumour refers to a metastasis from any mucus-secreting adenocarcinoma.

Meig syndrome may occur with a fibroma, Brenner tumour, thecoma or granulosa cell tumour.

CHAPTER 10

LEGAL ISSUES IN OBSTETRICS AND GYNAECOLOGY

> **Medical law and ethics are becoming increasingly important in all medical specialities, but especially in obstetrics and gynaecology. The rise in litigation in recent years has been dubbed a 'malpractice crisis'. Many obstetric claims receive large financial settlements and attract much media attention.**

CONSENT

Under common law it is well recognized that every person has the right to protect their bodily integrity against invasion by others. As a general rule, medical treatment, even of a minor nature, should not proceed unless the doctor has first obtained the patient's consent. Failure to do so may constitute battery (assault in Scotland), leading to civil claims, criminal prosecution or disciplinary procedures. The only two exceptions to obtaining consent are in an emergency situation, or with an unconscious patient.

Consent may be implied (e.g. rolling up a sleeve for a blood test) or expressed (orally or in writing). What needs to be disclosed remains a topic of intense legal and ethical debate. Many patients will want to know the potential problems in great detail, others will want only the minimum of information. It might be more relevant to warn a 30-year-old obese patient seeking a hysterectomy for menstrual problems about the risks of venous thromboembolic disease, for example, than to cover excessive detail about potential bowel injury in an otherwise well 50-year-old woman with well-differentiated endometrial carcinoma going for the same operation.

This would argue against general 'tick lists', although there may be a role for these in some instances (e.g. sterilization). Indeed, the issue of consent has assumed a significant place in the medical negligence debate in recent years, especially in claims for female sterilization. Some would argue that the minimum information disclosed should be the 'prudent patient' standard, i.e. what the patient thinks she should be told, whilst others argue that it should be the 'professional' standard, i.e. what the doctor thinks the patient should be told. The patient should be informed as fully as possible about the nature and consequences of treatment, and alternative therapies available, in a manner which the patient comprehends.

MEDICAL NEGLIGENCE

Although there has been a marked increase in recent years in the number of litigation claims and value of financial awards, it is still very difficult to succeed in an action of medical negligence in the UK. Not only are there practical difficulties in linking the injury of the plaintiff (or pursuer in Scotland) to medical treatment but, in medical negligence cases, the courts still effectively allow the standard of care to be defined by the medical profession itself.

The seminal legal cases are those of Hunter vs Hanley in Scotland [Hunter vs Hanley 1955 SC 200] and the English case of Bolam [Bolam vs Friern Hospital Management Committee [1957] 2 All ER 118, [1957] 1 WLR 582.], both of which define the essence of medical negligence. The Bolam dictum states, 'a doctor is not negligent if he acts in accordance with a practice accepted at the time as proper by a responsible body of medical opinion'. This is applicable not only to diagnosis and treatment but also the giving of information.

If a patient suffers harm as a result of treatment in hospital she may bring action for damages against the hospital. Vicarious liability means that the Trust is liable for any errors made by the doctor in the course of his or her employment.

For an action of medical negligence to succeed the patient must be able to show three things:

- The doctor owed the patient a duty of care.
- The doctor was in breach of that duty (i.e. failed to provide care of an adequate standard).
- The patient suffered harm as a consequence of that breach.

The burden of proof lies with the patient pursuing a claim of negligence. It is for the patient to show that, on the balance of probabilities, the doctor failed to meet the standard of care expected.

CONFIDENTIALITY

The requirement to protect patient confidentiality has long been included in the ethical codes of healthcare professionals (e.g. the Hippocratic oath). Protecting patient confidentiality may give rise to some very difficult moral and legal dilemmas (e.g. young girls requesting contraception, HIV testing in pregnancy).

There are exceptions to the confidentiality rule (General Medical Council). These include emergency situations, if the health or safety of the others are placed at serious risk, or if it is felt to be in the patient's best interests for confidentiality to be breached. Patients should always be told before confidentiality is breached.

FETOMATERNAL CONFLICT

Modern technology such as ultrasound scanning, which permits visualization of the fetus in utero, has led many to view the fetus as a person and patient, separate from the pregnant woman. This may create fetomaternal conflict, when the interests of the mother appear to diverge from those of the fetus.

Recent cases of court-authorized caesarean sections have highlighted the difficulties faced by doctors when a pregnant woman refuses to accept treatment which is thought by medical staff to be in the best interests of either herself or her baby. These judgments from the High Court which sanctioned the performance of caesarean sections against the mother's wishes received strong criticism for two main reasons.

- They contradict the generally held principle of the right to self-determination (autonomy). Many legal cases have demonstrated that, provided a patient has sufficient mental capability to understand the treatment options available they have the right to refuse treatment, even if it endangers their own life.
- It has been established in both the civil and criminal law that the fetus is not a person with legal rights and, as such, the courts do not have the power to protect the fetus.

The Court of Appeal subsequently reviewed these cases and concluded that it is unlawful to perform a caesarean section against a woman's wishes, if she is mentally competent. It is recommended that problem cases should be identified and brought before the courts early. There should be evidence, preferably from a psychiatrist, as to the woman's background and her mental capacity, and she should be legally represented in court. Doctors are under a duty to respect an advanced directive (i.e. expressed in advance of the emergency) from a competent patient refusing consent (e.g. one cannot perform a caesarean section against the patient's wishes if an advanced directive has been given against caesarean).

IF SOMETHING GOES WRONG

Most procedures carry recognized complications, despite being carried out by the most skilful and experienced operator. If complications arise they should be taken seriously, appropriately managed and the patient and relatives should be fully informed. Advice from senior colleagues should be sought at an early stage. Even if it is felt that an error has been made by somebody else, it is unwise to criticize another healthcare professional in front of the patient, particularly if the full facts are not yet known. However, if a mistake has been made, it is good practice to admit it and apologize to the patient personally. This does not imply negligence. Indeed, failure to disclose the error, provide information, and offer an apology increase the risk of litigation.

Medicine can never be free of mishaps. In our current medical culture, in which 'error' is often equated with 'incompetence', admission of errors to patients or fellow professionals is difficult. However, with clinical governance becoming an increasingly important aspect of healthcare, it is essential that mistakes are acknowledged and lessons learnt to prevent avoidable errors occurring again. Nobody is perfect, and not everybody owns a retrospectoscope.

DEFENSIVE PRACTICE

On of the genuine risks of increasing litigation is that we will act defensively, increase intervention and thereby *increase* morbidity and mortality. This defensiveness is not surprising as 70% of UK litigation relates to obstetrics, and the bill runs to billions of pounds. Most obstetric cases relate to labour ward practice, and 99% of these relate to 'failure to intervene' or 'delay in intervention'. Few cases are brought because of 'unnecessary intervention'.

As perinatal mortality is reduced and medical science becomes increasingly sophisticated, public expectations change. There is a tendency to believe that most, if not all deaths could have been prevented. Although confidential enquiries repeatedly show that suboptimal care is a serious problem contributing to preventable deaths, death is probably unavoidable in some mothers and babies. The courts are not always good at distinguishing between preventable and unavoidable deaths, and we must be careful to guard against the genuine risks to mothers and babies from defensive practice. If the growing trend towards medicalization is to be halted and reversed, the 'blame and claim' culture must be addressed (BMJ 2002;892). Childbirth without fear should become a reality for women, midwives, and obstetricians.

BPD (mm)	Gestation (weeks)
18	12+1
19	12+3
20	12+4
21	12+6
22	13+1
23	13+2
24	13+4
25	13+6
26	14+1
27	14+3
28	14+5
29	14
32	15
35	16
38	17
42	18
46	19
49	20
52	21
55	22

BPD (mm)	Gestation (weeks)
58	23
61	24
64	25
68	26
71	27
74	28
77	29
80	30
83	31
85	32
87	33
89	34
91	35
92	36
94	37
95	38
96	39
97	40
98	41
99	42

Appendix 1 Biparietal diameter.

CRL (mm)	−2 SD	Gestation (weeks)	+2 SD
6	6+1	7+1	8+0
7	6+3	7+2	8+2
8	6+4	7+4	8+3
9	6+6	7+6	8+6
10	7+1	8+0	9+0
11	7+2	8+2	9+1
12	7+3	8+3	9+3
13	7+5	8+4	9+4
14	7+6	8+6	9+6
15	8+0	9+0	10+0
16	8+2	9+2	10+1
17	8+3	9+3	10+2
18	8+4	9+4	10+4
19	8+5	9+5	10+5
20	8+6	9+6	10+6
21	9+0	10+0	11+0
22	9+1	10+1	11+1
23	9+2	10+2	11+2
24	9+3	10+3	11+3
26	9+5	10+5	11+5
28	9+6	11+0	12+1
30	10+1	11+2	12+2
32	10+2	11+3	12+4
34	10+4	11+5	12+5
36	10+5	11+6	13+0
38	10+6	12+1	13+2
40	11+1	12+2	13+3
42	11+2	12+3	13+4
44	11+3	12+4	13+6
46	11+5	12+6	14+0
48	11+6	13+0	14+2
50	11+6	13+1	14+3

Appendix 2 Crown–rump length (CRL).

Gestation from LMP (weeks)	Approx. sac on TV scan diameter (mm)	Earliest findings on TV scan	Earliest findings on TA scan
5.5	55	Sac	
5.5	58	FH and fetal pole	Sac
6.5	13		
6.5	17		FH and fetal pole
7.5	23		
8.5	32		
9.5	40		

Appendix 3 First trimester USS findings.

Appendix 4 Bi-parietal diameter: 5th, 50th and 95th centiles.

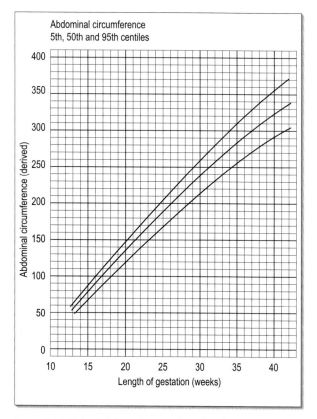

Appendix 5 Abdominal circumference: 5th, 50th and 95th centiles.

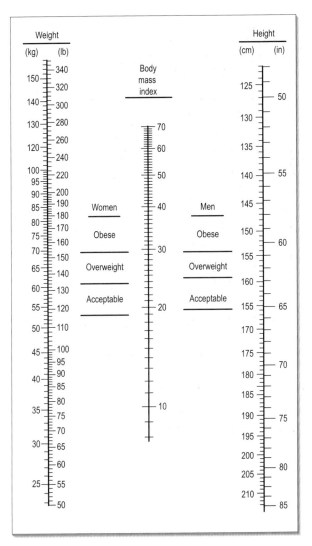

Appendix 6 Body mass index.